Robert,

the loving in your heart
spilled over and out
touching mine.
thank you for being my
teacher
I love you.

Jessica

THE LOVING DIET

❤

JESSICA FLANIGAN

THE

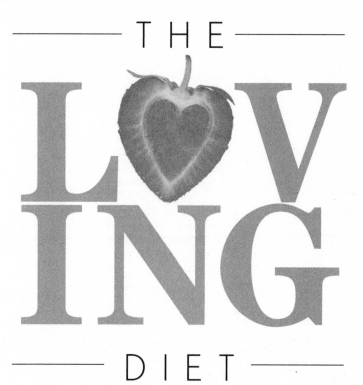

LOV ING

DIET

GOING BEYOND PALEO INTO
THE HEART OF WHAT AILS YOU

A POST HILL PRESS BOOK
ISBN: 978-1-61868-866-8
ISBN (eBook): 978-1-61868-867-5

THE LOVING DIET
Going Beyond Paleo into the Heart of What Ails You
© 2015 by Jessica Flanigan
All Rights Reserved

Cover Design by Diana Nuhn

Some names and situations have been changed or altered.

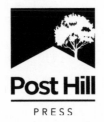

Post Hill Press
275 Madison Avenue, 14th Floor
New York, NY 10016
http://posthillpress.com

To my teacher Robert,
who showed me the way to love.

CONTENTS

INTRODUCTION

We are all here taking
the journey of love.

❤

OUR RELATIONSHIP TO OUR illness is the cure.

What is your relationship to your illness? Are you a victim? Is it hostile? Is it an unhappy relationship? You might not be able to change your illness, but you are completely capable of changing your relationship to your illness to create more happiness in your life. When you identify with loving instead of the pain, liberation, abundance, and joy are more available to you. The relationship to your illness then becomes one of cooperation. This book is going to show you that the remedy to what ails you is always loving and whatever form it takes, even as it relates to illness.

To achieve this relationship of cooperation, I'd like to ask you to consider a different way of living on this planet. It's not going to be easy; in fact, what I'm going to ask of you will at first be a more difficult approach than the one you're probably currently taking. But if you'll at least do your best to try, especially if you or someone you live with is suffering from an autoimmune disease or another serious health issue, I promise that you'll at least find peace despite the illness, and hopefully you'll find happiness. You might even find healing. Many of my clients have.

Doing so means you will have to make the decision to trust your life. Not many of us can wrap our heads around that notion and the challenges that it presents, but once you do—once you fully appreciate that there could be something bigger than each of us that is leading the world in which we live—you will see and experience dramatic change. Whatever it is—God, Buddha, The Divine—you'll come to understand and believe that this force may actually have your best interests in mind. And, if you don't believe in God, that is okay, too. Believe in love at least. Believing in love is somewhat central to The Loving Diet, so if you don't believe in love, you may hit a roadblock. But if you have ever loved something, someone, or felt what you considered a feeling of love, then that is enough. As long as you can recall that feeling, you will be able to produce the feelings of love for the exercises in this book.

The trust part might be more difficult. It's a tough notion to grasp, let alone live by. It means you're suddenly going to accept natural disaster or a cancer diagnosis. It means that you consider the idea that everything was and is supposed to happen the way it unfolds. It means that you use every situation in your life as an opportunity to grow. This is a noble idea, I'm aware, and perhaps until you embrace it, it's not going to make much sense to you, but once you do, it will all become clear.

If you're reading this right now, you want to take preventative action to find and maintain health and happiness, you are experiencing a significant life struggle, or you've hit rock bottom in terms of coping with your illness—whatever it is. That's when most of my clients reach out to me: once they've bottomed out. They've tried everything their various doctors have suggested and they may have even strictly followed the Autoimmune Paleo Diet protocol. Still, they're struggling, and they are miserable. That's because while they have adjusted their diet and understand the science of their medical diagnosis, they haven't yet considered a third prong to healing. It's the most critical component of all. It's the crux of The Loving Diet. It's the *loving* part. It's about taking the approach that the very thing that is afflicting us is doing so for our benefit. It is about mindfulness and meditation. It is about trusting that we can learn to lift ourselves up in our lives during the most challenging situations. It's the part that helps you come into cooperation with your illness and struggle. It's the part that takes you beyond eating Paleo—using a food diet similar to the Autoimmune Paleo food regimen as one component, and the science of your disease, and then adds in the healing benefits of mind and soul as well. The Loving Diet is a roadmap toward healing that will guide you to trust your life and learn to appreciate the struggle. Once you find peace, alignment will follow. It's based on love and all that love yields.

It may sound confusing or counterintuitive, or maybe even impossible to believe, but I know from experience that it works. I've built my practice on its proven success. I have taken the same path I ask my clients (and am asking you) to trust themselves to take. I did not happen upon my path from disease. But does it really matter how we hear the call of our hearts, as long as we do? We all have a language we recognize inside ourselves that calls us to attention in life. My call to attention was a matter of the heart. I have deeply suffered. I suspect you are suffering now, too.

A "CHARMED" LIFE

I had what anyone would classify as a perfect life. From the outside my husband and I had everything: house, cars, community, and success. I had built a fantastic life to hide from myself. My husband and I had been together for a decade. We were not really happy, but I didn't know how unhappy I was because I was so busy choosing safety and security. In doing so, I tuned out everything else. I thought I was experiencing the normal level of unhappiness many marriages experience as couples attempt to manage so much. We were married at thirty-one, had a baby at thirty-two, were successful business owners at thirty-three, and bought our dream house at thirty-five. I would have remained in the unhappy, stressful place indefinitely because I was too scared to leave.

I knew I was unhappy because I never felt fulfilled. I felt a constant drive inside of myself for more. I felt anxious most of the time. I almost obsessively worried about my health. When I had time alone, I felt sad. I kept thinking I would feel happy when I reached the next goal. Each time I reached a goal (baby, career, house, status), I would cross the finish line and look around and feel let down when life remained the same. The goals got bigger, the stakes higher, and all the while the pressure increased. I placed tremendous pressure on my husband to perform for the family, so we could continue achieving and looking like the superstar couple who lived in the modern house on the meadow. Secretly, my husband and I were miserable, without a vocabulary to express it. Neither of us was happy. We argued frequently, and the resentment kept building over time. Even couples therapy did not seem to help.

We lacked the tools to change our happiness level. I would randomly buy self-help books and try to find a secret formula. I went to see a therapist and I had energy work done. I meditated. I searched long and hard and long and hard for those tools to make life happier, better. How this translated to my everyday life: I tried to control nearly everything. I became almost obsessive about germs and sickness. For example, I would leave parties early if there were sick children present. I kept hand sanitizer on me at all times. I would not eat food at my friends' potlucks for fear of food poisoning. I became convinced that I knew the right way to do things when it came to eating, cooking, cleaning, and socializing. I was pretty regimented. I had crystal-clear definitions of right and wrong. Surely being right would guide me to more happiness, right?

Wrong, actually. It was all compensation for something else.

There was a deeper place inside of me that was terrified to be responsible for my own life. Terrified of change. Terrified that change would push me into a void and my life would be even more miserable. I would dream about being on vacation all the time. Then, when I was actually on vacation, I would be scared the entire time that I would get sick and my vacation would be ruined. I never seemed to set up a win-win scenario for myself. What I did not know was that deep down I held a belief that I did not deserve a win-win. That should have been a clue for something deeper at play. I did not really think I deserved health, wealth, and happiness. And yet, it was the very thing I strove for, plotted for, dreamed about, and constantly searched for every day. If my fate was unhappiness, at least I would be unhappy in a nice house. I was determined to sit tight and keep creating happiness on the outside to convince my inside that I was happy. If my life appeared perfect enough, eventually I would feel complete and happy. I was certain. I wanted change and I had no idea how to achieve it. I wanted to be happy and I attempted every effort to attain it. I searched out healers (when I should have been finding teachers), meditated, was kind to others, perfected throwing dinner parties, became class parent at my daughter's school, took vitamins, got acupuncture, did yoga. . . . The list goes on and on.

> There was a deeper place inside of me that was terrified to be responsible for my own life.

LIFE HAD OTHER PLANS

One of the worst scenarios I could have imagined of my life falling apart became a reality. My husband met someone while commuting to the Bay Area. He arrived home one day and told me he wanted to end our marriage. He moved out the next day, three hours away, to live with the other woman. I was left to crumble (which I did) with a six-year-old, a house, and a community of people who felt the shockwave of the "most solid couple" suddenly splitting. We had had such a public life that the phone started ringing and the naturally curious wanted to know the *whats* and the *whys*. I immediately gathered my close friends, turned off the phone, got off the Internet, and promptly and completely fell apart. *Like really fell apart.* I went into a complete state of shock and grief. The only way I can describe it was feeling like I had been pushed off a cliff. I spent days crying and unable to move. I sat in the bathtub for hours every night sobbing. And yet, I had been so unhappy for so long that a deeper part of me was not surprised. But still, I remained in a deep pool of sadness, anger, confusion, and humiliation. And I stayed there for more than a year. Then we lost our house. We had built it at the top of the market and then we were suddenly under water after the market crashed. I fumbled, trying to take care of a young child when all I wanted to do was cry all day. I felt the embarrassment from being known as the scorned woman, left for a younger one. Life was not unfolding in the magical way I'd hoped. It was actually imploding.

But grace was with me the entire time, as it is with you, too. Early in the split, I sat down one night and had a conversation with the Divine. I told God I would trust my life and trust that this disaster had my best interests in mind. I had become hip to the fact that I needed something a bit more powerful than therapy and self-help books, and I asked the wisest person I know, my teacher and mentor Robert, how I could possibly get through my life falling apart. He said, "You have to believe you will wash up on dry shore." And so I did. I sat down and decided to tell God I would trust this. And while this commitment did not ease my suffering, it did at least give me a focus. Every day I would wake up (and start crying, wishing I could remain indefinitely in the sleep state rather than deal with the bone-chilling grief that came in powerful waves day after day) and repeat over and over again: *I trust my life.*

One day, about nine months after the ceiling of life fell down on me, I was having a session with a healer. She suggested I love the grief. I was so struck by how backward and yet aligned that statement sounded. I had been suffering for so many months at that point that I was willing to try anything to make the pain go away. I remember feeling so tired of being sad that I was willing to give loving grief a shot. I lay down in my bed and said, "Okay, grief, I love you. Do whatever you want." And I let go. Really, really let go. I let go and I wondered if I might lose my mind, because I had just given grief permission to come in and take over my life. I cried, not from sadness in that moment but from fear that I was willingly letting go of every molecule of control and instead trusting something to come forward without any assurance of a safe outcome. For the very first time, I let go and trusted my life. And if it fell apart, so be it. I was so tired of trying and surviving, fighting and coping. And for the whole night I lay there and felt the experience of something else purposing my life and the scary and new feeling of taking my hands off the steering wheel I had gripped so tightly.

ENTER LOVE

The next day I woke up and took a shower. I do believe it was the first shower I had taken in months during which I did not cry. And I managed to make dinner that next night. I remember the feeling of relaxation washing over me like I had never experienced before, due to the feeling of loving my grief. I loved the sad me over those next days and months. I took sad me to the movies. I took her to the grocery store. I did not try to be anywhere but in the sad place. And that was when I began to feel better. I stopped trying to fight change. I stopped the fighting, period. I acknowledged that I knew nothing about how to be a happy person, and I stopped judging myself for feeling so ignorant about it. I just allowed myself to feel the feeling of being lost. I started to feel very humble. I stopped planning how my grief would end. I just stopped. I stopped everything, except eating, sleeping, and parenting. The crying lessened. The pain lessened.

When I stopped fighting so hard *against* life not being what I wanted or thought, I had longer and longer stretches without crying. Eventually, as I gathered my strength, I had to face the fact that blaming anyone else for my circumstances wasn't useful for my own growth. That was hard. Blaming my husband and his girlfriend made me feel better. It took the pressure off me to be responsible for my mess. It was so much more difficult to look at myself. I had to face facts that I was the sole author of my story. But here is the key: *I had decided to love the grief.* And in my dedication to trusting my life and loving the grief, an amazing upside started to surface. Life falling apart did not equal life falling apart. Life meant trusting that every single little thing that was happening to me was for my benefit. And even though I had no idea what the benefit might be, I just kept trusting it. The suffering, pain, loss, and grief all had a secret message of hope and love. All were coming forward to help me love myself, love my crumbled life, love how I was managing my pain, and love the fear of not knowing how life would unfold. I started forgiving myself for the regret that I had stayed in my marriage for so long, forgiving the people I thought were hurting me, and forgiving myself when I did become mean and belittling to my ex and his girlfriend.

I just stopped trying and I started loving.

Now, I am able to trust life so deeply that it is my spiritual practice. Loving is my method. I love what is here, no matter what costume it is wearing. If someone is mean, I love them. If someone rejects me, I love that, too. Because I know in the core of my being that nothing comes present in life unless it has something to teach me for my soul's growth. This of course doesn't mean I don't suffer or feel sad. This means that when *bad* things happen now, I take a perspective that there is a deeper purpose for it coming forward than a bad deal or disruption. It comes forward because it can help me grow deeper into my life and a loving state.

Illness may be the vehicle for you, the way heartbreak was for me. I do believe illness can be the messenger for happiness and joy for us if *we choose it* to be so. I do believe that disruption of any kind actually is here to help us, free us, and love us. And when we consider that option inside of us, then life becomes that on the outside of us. This path took its time unfolding itself to me. It was not an overnight process. It was a gradual process that has gained momentum in the last few years. I took this journey inch by inch, at first. But now I take the perspective that there is no such thing as *good* or *bad*. There is only more to experience that will assist me with loving everything. There are only experiences that deepen my inner foundation to trust, love, and grow. Happiness comes to me in unlimited amounts now by trusting my life.

My divorce became final four years after we split. I was so sad for so long that I could not face going through the legal process any sooner. Eventually, however, I came so far with my grief and my relationship with my ex-husband that I moved to the same town as him and his girlfriend. And I am proud and happy to report we are all friends. I have a tremendous amount of gratitude for their love, patience, and understanding. I feel deep gratitude that they helped me discover the happiness I had been searching for my whole life. I have a genuine, heartfelt want for their happiness. They are part of how I got the life I have now that I love so much. They are part of the story that helped The Loving Diet modality to come forward. They are loving teachers. When I stopped judging how my story was unfolding, I was able to love them both and appreciate the humanness we all have. I sit in complete honor of all the souls who help me grow and love more. Nothing is an obstacle. Anything that I think is in my way or blocking me is a gift of growth. A secret whisper that will allow more loving into my life.

If I choose it.

BEYOND PALEO: COMBINING LOVE WITH SCIENCE

There's more to my path of loving as well—the science and the nutrition. I initially embraced the Autoimmune Paleo Diet (AIP) when my twin sister was diagnosed with two autoimmune diseases. I, therefore, have a 75 percent chance of having the same genetics. That puts me at risk for having celiac disease and for having Hashimoto's thyroiditis. In the search for answers for us both, we started looking into our genetic history. We're fairly certain our grandmother had celiac, our grandfather had psoriasis, and our father has Hashimoto's. I began practicing as well as teaching the AIP diet to prevent the genes from getting turned on. We know that if you have the autoimmunity genes and you have a really horrible virus or a major stress event, it can turn them on.

I did a ton of detective work, in part because it took my sister two years to get diagnosed and in part because of my pre-disposition, considering my family history. I went on a fact-finding mission, learning the benefits of Autoimmune Paleo eating for those struggling, like my sister, and those like me who could potentially struggle and are therefore pre-emptively embracing the protocol.

I combined my seventeen years of work as a functional clinical nutritionist specializing in AIP with my ten years' experience with the science behind the benefits of being mindful and my discovery of the benefits of loving to create The Loving Diet. It's been a continually evolving and growing practice for me, but I've been moved and overwhelmed by how many people reach out in need of what I can offer. Thousands of people visit my website each month, mostly desperate for guidance. I run monthly workshops across the country to give some hands-on and group guidance, in addition to operating my practice in Northern California. My clients teach me as much as I teach them. So I decided to try to capture all of it here—I've collected all of the experience and developed a plan that is self-guided. It's for those who need my guidance but want to or must work on their own from home. There are multiple resources to aid you as you work through this book, including my websites, AIPLifestyle.com and TheLovingDiet.com, and other products that will help you. There are outside resources listed at the end of the book, too. But within these pages rests all of my work so you can hopefully live the benefits from home on your own. I do suggest pairing up with a nutritionist or a Loving Diet practitioner if you can afford one. Consult your doctor as well for resources.

In addition to the loving element, I'm going to show you how to eat my modified version of the AIP protocol, which helps heal the immune system. Many of you may have already started some variation of AIP or Paleo but may now be discovering it isn't quite enough. One in six people get an autoimmune disease in his or her life, and for many, in my opinion, the gateway autoimmune disease—Hashimoto's disease—sets one up to develop more in his or her lifetime. I have my clients follow AIP to reduce inflammation in the intestines—the driving force of autoimmune disease, after all, has its beginning roots in the gut. The food diet aspect is similar to AIP, or at least that's the foundation, but it extends beyond that both in food intake and in loving—coming into cooperation with an illness. My clients have at the very least found happiness and peace through The Loving Diet, and many report an alleviation of their symptoms. When we come into cooperation through loving what ails us, we create an opportunity in both our body and mind for healing. I have found that love and loving our challenges is the most rapid form of change both in our hearts and lives. When we develop skills to increase self-compassion and tenderness toward ourselves and our circumstances, life transforms itself to meet us with joy, abundance, and health. For many people, this can create leaps in their health journey. For others, it is a calm acceptance that creates more space for joy.

THE LOVING DIET

The Loving Diet will both help you assess your illness and make it an ally rather than an obstacle and teach you to eat in a way that aligns you with your healing and inner teacher. You'll completely alter your relationship with your disease. You may not realize it just yet, but you already have all the tools inside of you to come into cooperation with your illness. You just need to tap into them. That is really the secret sauce. It is not a *doing* process to increase happiness and health; it is an *awakening* process. Awakening to the idea that everything that happens in life is here to help your life in some way, including illness. When you start investing in the idea of trusting your life, you will tap into an understanding that the illness you're living with might just have a positive aspect to it: wisdom.

Remember, the illness is just there, like the person who came to the party uninvited. I always think the uninvited guest is the one who possibly has the best jokes—the illness may have your best interests in mind. If even for a moment you can consider the idea that the illness has something to give instead of take away, then it is instantly working in your favor. Then life opens up as a series of opportunities and it becomes your decision each time if you are going to take off the ugly costume and see what riches lie inside. Even if it means your life falls apart, it is doing so because wisdom is trying to come forward in the process. Then use the struggle and the willingness to your advantage. Those things can come forward through the doing and trying, too, but in some ways it is like making our bag of tricks in life include all of what makes us up, not just the "good" stuff. I think this is far more rewarding because then you don't have to discount anything in life. Then the messed up childhoods, bad marriages, tragedies, and diseases all get starring roles in our greatness, not just the awards, grand houses, or big incomes. Think about that for a minute. We are all trying to run away from the things that we don't like, or others don't like, in ourselves and trying to be perfect. But the imperfections are opportunities for being vulnerable, building courage, and ultimately increasing wisdom. We choose to decide if we will love them. And when we do, when we love the difficulties in our life, they open a door to the idea that we are already whole and perfect, and adversity was just the way we came to understand that truth.

It was through heartbreak that I eventually chose love. I chose me and believing in me. And I chose trusting that I could do it. And I know you can, too. And while illness may be your vehicle and not heartbreak, I believe in you. I really, really believe in you.

THE HAPPINESS QUIZ

Grab a notebook and answer *yes* or *no* to the following questions:

1. Do you wake up interested in your life?
2. Do you regularly have time for yourself each week?
3. When you are by yourself, do you feel happy?
4. Do you depend on yourself for happiness as opposed to your closest relationships?
5. Are you able to avoid eating to make yourself feel better?

If you answered *no* to three or more of these questions, you may need to look a bit deeper at your happiness level. Keep reading. I'm going to help you do so. You can trust what's coming forward—you won't be in this place forever. The unhappiness can motivate you to find something more. That's wisdom. Start thinking about your resources: your therapist, inspirations, friends, doctors, healing practitioners, and this book. Then, I'm going to ask you to create a new roadmap to healing by accepting within yourself the place that isn't happy, and by having a willingness to change. Also, by drawing upon the resources you already have and knowing that ultimately you are okay. Sometimes the road to being happy is through unhappiness—like with illness. Don't disregard the unhappiness caused by your illness. It might just be the ticket to your happy place.

A LOVING AFFIRMATION

Take one step toward coming into cooperation with your illness. Wake up each morning and say, "I trust my life."

PART
1

MEDICAL

Healing is the journey we take

to believe we are worth our

own fearlessness.

1

WHAT IS AUTOIMMUNE DISEASE?

Loving is the truth.

💜

THE LOVING DIET IS for anyone who is struggling or knows someone who is struggling. While the notion behind it will aid the healing process for any disease, and eventually other aspects of your life, such as love, your career, and goals, the majority of my clients have one or more autoimmune diseases. That's been the foundation of my work as a nutritionist and mind-body practitioner. Since the food portion of The Loving Diet protocol has its roots in the Autoimmune Paleo eating protocol, I wanted to start with some background information on autoimmune disease, so that you fully understand its impact on the body and know the signs.

AUTOIMMUNE DISEASE

Autoimmune disease (AD) occurs when the body's cells get confused. The immune system, which protects the body against disease, starts attacking and damaging healthy tissue. It's a common disease—one in six people in the United States suffers from it. Worse, we know that it is on the rise. The National Institutes of Health estimates that 23.5 million people in the United States have AD. In comparison, cancer affects nine million people.

Heart disease: 22 million.[1] The American Autoimmune Related Disease Association (AARDA) estimates that closer to 50 million people suffer from it. Theoretically, a mixture of genetics, environmental pollutants, viruses, and stress in some combination turns on the autoimmune genes. According to the New York Academy of Sciences,[2] environmental factors are generally considered the culprits for how quickly AD progresses as well as for the loss of integrity in the intestinal epithelium. Increased permeability in the intestines always precedes autoimmune disease.

When the body cannot distinguish between healthy tissue and foreign invaders and a hypersensitive reaction occurs, it starts self-tissue attack. For months, or perhaps years, this self-tissue attack can occur silently until full-blown autoimmune disease develops. According to the AARDA, there are more than eighty to one hundred types of "official" autoimmune disorders (and *many* more are being discovered daily), but all autoimmune diseases share the symptoms of tissue self-attacking in places like the thyroid gland, brain tissue, or salivary glands, to name a few. Inflammation in the small intestine is now suspected of being one of the physiological dysfunctions related to autoimmune disease. Inflammation in the small intestine can be caused from small intestinal bacterial overgrowth (SIBO), food sensitivities and allergies, viruses, environmental toxins, hormones, parasites, and stress. Inflammation in the small intestine tends to be the beginnings of the physiological dysfunction related to autoimmune disease. From there, a ripple effect takes place.

CAUSES OF AUTOIMMUNE DISEASE

Autoimmune diseases have their roots in genetics. You may never express it, but you might have genes for type 1 diabetes or another illness. We now know that gene expression can be caused by one of the following factors:

---

1 www.aarda.org/autoimmune-information/autoimmune-statistics.
2 www.ncbi.nlm.nih.gov/pmc/articles/PMC2886850/.

- Illness
- Stress
- Inflammation
- Environmental pollutants

If anything feels out of the ordinary with your body—numbness, weight gain, swelling, tingling, hair loss, or any number of symptoms—you need to be under a doctor's care. Most allopathic treatment models include immune suppressant drugs. Functional medicine tends to take a different approach by looking at inflammation that drives autoimmunity.[3]

TYPES OF AUTOIMMUNE DISEASE[4]

There are two types of autoimmune disease: organ specific and non–organ specific.

There's also overlap and some diseases land in between.

Organ-specific diseases include:

- Hashimoto's thyroiditis (thyroid gland)
- Pernicious anemia (stomach)
- Addison's disease (adrenal glands)
- Type 1 diabetes (pancreas)

Non–Organ-specific diseases include:

- Rheumatoid arthritis
- Systemic lupus erythematosus
- Dermatomyositis

There are so many types of AD, I couldn't begin to list them all or identify every one for you, but the most common among my clients is

---

3 http://drhyman.com/blog/2010/10/09/is-there-a-cure-for-autoimmune-disease/.

4 www.aarda.org/autoimmune-information/questions-and-answers/.

Hashimoto's disease, so I will provide some in-depth information here, since it is likely the most common disease among readers.

HASHIMOTO'S DISEASE: POTENTIAL GATEWAY TO OTHER AUTOIMMUNE DISEASES?

Hypothyroidism occurs when an underactive thyroid gland does not produce enough thyroid hormone. Ninety percent of all women who have hypothyroidism get Hashimoto's disease in their lifetime.[5]

Hashimoto's disease is defined by medical science as being hypothyroid and having the presence of thyroid antibody. Once that signaling gets turned on in someone's body where that tissue self-attack occurs, then the propensity for that tissue self-attack on the immune system increases, and the body starts attacking healthy tissue and other parts of the body as well. Once autoimmune disease is identified, the likelihood of being diagnosed with additional autoimmune diseases increases.

Ninety percent of all women who have hypothyroidism get Hashimoto's in their lifetime.

♥

Common symptoms of Hashimoto's disease include:

- Hair loss
- Inability to regulate body temperature
- Weight gain or weight loss

---

5 www.ncbi.nlm.nih.gov/pubmed/3066320.

- Brain fog
- Digestive issues
- Dry skin
- Constipation

If you have a number of these symptoms, you should see a doctor and ask to have your thyroid antibodies tested.

THE STAGES OF AUTOIMMUNITY

There are three stages of autoimmunity generally recognized by alternative and functional medical practitioners, although not by traditional medicine. The blog HashimotosHealing.com has incredible information on dealing with autoimmune disease, in particular the discussion of its three stages.[6] As a practitioner, I try to be aware of the different stages my clients might encounter and the strategies to prevent entering the disease state. Also, I try to make sure they're going to see a doctor if they're experiencing stage-two symptoms.

STAGE 1: SILENT AUTOIMMUNITY

This stage marks the presence of tissue antibodies. Some people call them auto-antibodies—antibodies directed against the person who produced them. During this stage, you'll likely have no symptoms and would only know that you have an AD if you have lab work done. It's likely we all have tissue antibodies to a degree, but in many it remains benign. For others, it lays dormant for years before transitioning to disease state or a different stage.

---

6 www.hashimotoshealing.com/hashimotos-is-an-autoimmune-disease-so-why-is-everyone-ignoring-the-autoimmune-part/

STAGE 2: AUTOIMMUNE SYMPTOMS BEGIN

At this stage, the destruction of your tissue has already started. Your antibodies have elevated, but you have not developed what would be called full-blown autoimmune disease because not enough of your tissue has been destroyed. This is a critical stage. There's still potential to course-correct and heal. I hope this is the future of autoimmune disease right here: doctors who are willing to take it seriously when antibodies are detected in patients, but before a diagnosable disease manifests. Intervention here is critical. Both the Autoimmune Paleo Diet and The Loving Diet are tools that address the progression of inflammation, which may be implicated with moving from stage two into stage three of autoimmunity.

Symptoms of stage two include:

- Anything that makes a person not feel well or seems abnormal
- Pain of some kind or just an "off" feeling
- Physiological dysfunction such as fatigue, joint or muscle pain, numbness, tingling, skin issues, weight gain, weight loss, balance changes, and visual changes

What if somehow you recognize yourself in stage two? Perhaps you have pain and you make an appointment to see your doctor. You get tested thoroughly and come up positive for ANA antibodies, and your doctor tells you one of three things:

- "Don't worry about it."
- "Let's watch and see."
- "Nothing is wrong with you."

I encourage you to use this as critical information to thoughtfully form your health-care team and be more proactive. A positive ANA antibody, or any autoimmune antibody, should attract your attention and be taken seriously. Find people who will listen and help you make lifestyle changes to address the antibodies.

By the way, I see this frequently in my practice. It's often when people come to me for guidance. If you experience any of these symptoms, go to a doctor. If you don't feel you received answers, listen to yourself. If you don't like the answer your doctor has given you, look at your family history and get a second or third opinion. Find someone who will listen. Find someone who will test antibodies.

This stage is the opportunity stage. Find help. Continue to look. Your body is telling you something meaningful. Practice The Loving Diet.

STAGE 3: AUTOIMMUNE DISEASE

If you've reached this stage, it's very late in the game. You have full-blown autoimmune disease. Tests have revealed tissue damage and the presence of positive antibodies. At this point everything is being managed by doctors. Western medicine will have discovered and acknowledged the disease. They may or may not have ways to help you through medication, but that's the extent of what they can do: watch, manage, medicate. Now is the time for you to embrace The Loving Diet. It will give you information on eating a low-inflammatory diet and how to come into cooperation with your circumstances.

Common Autoimmune Diseases Include:

Graves' disease   Celiac disease

Multiple sclerosis   Psoriasis

Rheumatoid arthritis   Inflammatory bowel

Type 1 diabetes   disease

Lupus   Sjögren's syndrome

Hashimoto's disease

AUTOIMMUNE DISEASE AND SIBO: THE BASICS

Gut issues tend to go hand-in-hand with autoimmune disease. One doesn't cause the other, but one of the most common gut issues I see among my autoimmune population is small intestinal bacterial overgrowth (SIBO). SIBO is gaining a lot of traction in the functional medical field. Estimates show that up to 80 percent of those with irritable bowel syndrome have SIBO. Overgrowth of certain bacteria in the small intestine can be problematic for many and includes symptoms of gas, bloating, constipation, and abdominal pain.

Bacterial overgrowth in the small intestine is due to a migration of native large intestine bacteria to the small intestine for various reasons. Low stomach acid, low intestinal motility, and a stressful lifestyle are some of the causes. Illness (IBS, H. pylori, and celiac, to name a few) and chronic constipation may weaken the ileocecal valve, contributing to the migration of the microbial environment from the large to small intestine. These *out-of-place* bacteria then feed on the not-yet-digested foods found in the small intestine, grow in numbers, and create a host of physical and digestive disturbances known as SIBO.

Because the large intestine inherently has a larger population of bacteria in comparison to the small intestine, bacteria normally found in the colon takes up residence in the small intestine and causes profound changes, such as how well the small intestine can digest and absorb food, micronutrients, and amino acids. When bacteria migrate from the large to small intestine, the bacteria are exposed to different food sources in the form of starches, fibers, and sugars. These provide a rich environment for the misplaced bacteria, which then grow in numbers in the small intestine. This accelerated bacterial growth creates the symptoms we now associate with SIBO. Furthermore, certain probiotics and fermented foods can aggravate this situation and add to the problem of overgrowth.

Functionally, when the small intestine is overgrown with bacteria, it cannot perform its normal functions of absorption, but SIBO can also create or exacerbate issues of leaky gut. There is a way to help heal SIBO, however, although it can be a long and tricky path filled with repeated doses of antibiotics that may or may not work, a major diet adjustment (which alone is not enough), and simultaneous healing of the intestinal mucosa. Not all the treatments are effective, and some treatments need to be repeated. Working with a health-care practitioner is essential in this regard.

HOW TO TEST FOR SIBO

A breath test is the most up-to-date form of detecting SIBO. A sample of breath measures levels of hydrogen and methane. Different SIBO bacteria produce these gases in the small intestine. A breath test for SIBO may not be as accurate as we would like, but it is the best kind of testing available to date. Although false positives are rarer, false negatives are common. It is best to work with a practitioner to assess symptoms and use that as a benchmark for treatment along with a breath test.

For the most part, our body is equipped naturally to prevent SIBO. In many cases, however, there are potential causes and risk factors, such as:[7]

- Heavy to moderate alcohol use
- Birth control pills
- Crohn's disease
- Overuse of antibiotics
- Low stomach acid
- Irritable bowel syndrome
- Celiac disease
- Bowel surgery
- Type 1 and 2 diabetes
- Organ dysfunction
- Chronic constipation

---

7 www.chriskresser.com/.

- Certain medications
- GERD
- H. pylori infections

It's a challenge to diagnose SIBO. Testing is important, but I don't always rely on it 100 percent. A good practitioner is important to help you figure it out and heal it. SIBO, untreated, can be harmful. The gut is an important blood-brain barrier. SIBO is the failure and breakdown of that barrier. It's an important piece of the autoimmune puzzle.

❤ ❤ ❤

You likely already are experiencing much of what you just read about. Or you're suffering in another way—from cancer or a crisis. Find help and don't quit until you do. Trust how you're feeling and believe you can resolve it and create a plan for yourself.

2

DOCTORS AND TESTS

Your heart holds the healing.

💜

MODERN MEDICINE SAVES LIVES. That's not up for debate. That's a fact. My ex-husband is a Type 1 diabetic. If he didn't have insulin to manage his autoimmune disease, he wouldn't be alive. Think of all of the scenarios in which medicine has saved lives: C-sections, emergency appendix removal, antibiotics, chemotherapy, and open-heart surgery. This list is endless.

People become frustrated with their doctors and with traditional medicine because they don't feel better working with them. Often, they find alternate practitioners and start to ignore their doctor's orders, or they stop taking their medications. It's important that you don't do that: Do not take yourself off your medication. You have to work with your doctor when you are prescribed medicine. Discontinuing any prescribed medicine could make everything much, much worse.

To be clear, I'm by no means asking you to ignore modern medicine. In fact, I'm asking that you make it the third prong in The Loving Diet—working with doctors in conjunction with the mind-loving element and the food protocol. Still, that doesn't mean stop questioning.

Autoimmune disease is a chronic disease. In some cases, doctors don't have the skill to naturally treat it. That doesn't mean that they're ill-intentioned or that they don't care, but I've noticed that people who want to take a deeper look at their disease, like we are in this book, often move past the wall they've hit with a traditional doctor or are asking for more information than their doctors can offer.

I want to suggest to you a new approach to creating a health-care plan if you have been diagnosed with an autoimmune disease. It requires that you take some control, ask questions, and be in charge of your health care. Or even that you become a partner with your doctor. It might feel odd to question a doctor or change altogether if you don't feel okay with what you hear, but I want you to know you can. You know your body. You want to find someone who is aligned with your needs and gut reactions. Start with these three steps:

1. Always start with the question "Is this path the most loving to me?" Then begin hiring your team. It is important to keep in mind that you always have a choice and you get to hire (and fire if you need to) your whole team.
2. Doctors play a very important role in your health-care plan, and being sure that your team has your best interests at heart, listens well, and advocates for you is critical.
3. When you look at your team and start to build it from scratch, consider consulting more than just doctors, including:
   - Pharmacist: Your pharmacist is a wealth of information about drug interactions and ingredients.
   - Spiritual advisors (minister, priest, rabbi, guru): This person will help you put your disease in perspective and give you strength to work through the hurdles.
   - Alternative medical practitioner: A concrete and complete healing plan is important and, oftentimes, an alternative practitioner will round out that plan, adding to what a medical doctor will provide you with.
   - Friends and family: The day-in-day-out cheerleaders are important to your journey. Keep them informed and lean on them.

I want to suggest to you a new approach to creating a health-care plan if you have been diagnosed with an autoimmune disease. It requires that you take some control, ask questions, and be in charge of your health care.

HOW TO MANAGE YOUR DOCTOR

There was probably a time or an era when people went to the doctor and did what they were told without questioning the diagnosis or prescribed fixes. Today, things are a bit different. There are more alternatives available, probably more diseases and illness we know of, and more opportunity for you to be an active partner in your own health care. You may also have some flexibility to find the right doctor to fit your needs instead of sticking with one who doesn't.

If you're at the stage where you're completely frustrated and you've tried all the advice of your doctor, that's okay. Keep on it. Keep asking, keep pushing, keep finding a like-minded caregiver and practitioner. It's frustrating. You want to be heard and maybe you feel like you're not.

Having said that, I understand if you wind up going down the rabbit hole with a doctor who charges fees not covered by your insurance, who has had you buy supplements and prescriptions, and who has given you a battery of expensive tests. Still, you have to trust your gut and keep looking if you feel like it's not working. I suggest asking yourself continually "Is this the most loving path for me?" and seeing what develops. There's one way to ensure your practitioner is the right fit. It's almost like trusting that you're going to find the right people by having the intentions that you will. And as you make your way through all the prongs of The Loving Diet, perhaps a clearer picture of who can best help will emerge.

If you have a frustrating—or even bad—doctor, you just have to trust it and believe that whatever comes forward is meant to come forward. Every experience that we have has some kind of wisdom for our life, whether it be a bad experience or a good experience.

I tell people to find what and who resonates for them and their own personal philosophy. Sometimes, that is a medical doctor. Sometimes, it's a naturopath—a doctor who has medical training at a naturopathic medical university. Sometimes, it's an Asian medical doctor. Half of it is finding out what you feel aligned with and, when you find it, trusting it.

WHAT TO LOOK FOR IN YOUR PRACTITIONERS

- They let you ask questions.
- They continue to ask questions on your behalf.
- They have a true willingness for your health to improve.
- They don't put you down or discount your ideas and opinions.
- They freely admit when they don't know or understand something.
- They are open to working with others on your healthcare team.

MANAGING YOUR OWN MEDICINE

Start a file of everything relating to your disease, so that you can easily find all of your information when you need it.

- Get copies of everything, so that if you hop around or go to a specialist, you have all of the information at your fingertips.
- Don't leave your doctor's office without labs in hand.

■ You can do out-of-pocket testing at places like DirectLabs.com and others like it and then bring your labs to doctors until you get answers. See my Wellness Panel.

MY PERSONAL WELLNESS PANEL

Every year I do a battery of tests on myself. This list of tests looks at thyroid function, blood lipids, levels of iron in the blood, and general inflammatory markers. This blood work is my suggested starting place to truly find out your basic physiology. On Directlabs.com, this is called the APEX 5 Panel. You'll need a doctor or nutritionist to interpret the results. Here's my list:

Comprehensive Metabolic Panel w/ eGFR
Complete Blood Count w/ Differential
C-Reactive Protein
Ferritin
Hemoglobin A1c
VLDL (very low density lipoprotein)
TIBC (total iron binding capacity)
% Iron Saturation
Serum Iron
Sedimentation Rate
TSH (thyroid stimulating hormone)
T3 (triiodothyronine)
T3 Uptake
T4 Thyroxine Total
T4 Thyroxine Free
Reverse T3
Free T3
Uric Acid
1,25- Dihydroxy Vitamin D

continued

Thyroid Peroxidase (TPO) Antibodies

Thyroglobulin Antibodies

Homocysteine

Standard Urinalysis

I also do a stool test, a cortisol saliva test, and antibody testing on myself.

Unless you live in New York or New Jersey, you can order lab work yourself online and pay for it out of pocket, which I find more and more people are really willing to do now, out of desperation. They can then bring their lab work to practitioners who can translate this kind of lab work to look at their health and nutritional status, not just looking for disease like many doctors do.

DON'T GIVE UP

Even if you've reached rock bottom in terms of being heard and finding help, remember why you're reading this: You're searching for answers and you haven't been able to find them. This book will help you take a deeper look at your healing resources, especially if you've tried many things that haven't worked.

The Loving Diet will remind you:

- You can do this.
- There's a good reason why this is happening.
- There's a deeper meaning behind the illness.
- Love is ultimately the driving force behind our lives and all our experiences

Caregivers can benefit from reading this, too. They fall into a role as well, because sometimes when we are sick we get hopeless, and so we look to the people that we love for hope. I really want this book to offer hope that there is more than medicines to help our bodies heal.

If it helps, keep a medicine journal. Or check your phone or computer. There is, as they say, "an app for that." Keep all of your information together as you seek answers.

3

SCIENCE NOW REVEALS MINDFULNESS MATTERS

Trust your life.

♥

*J*anice felt badly for years. She had no energy, was depressed, and had horrible brain fog, chronic stomachaches and bloating, and mysterious hair loss. At first she thought she was just getting old. After seeing three doctors, she finally found an integrative medical doctor who ran the right tests and confirmed her symptoms were not in her head but sadly she had in fact developed two autoimmune diseases. Janice was diagnosed with Hashimoto's and celiac disease. Upon diagnosis, she fell into a depression and also lost her job.

Janice decided to start The Loving Diet after reading about the Autoimmune Paleo Diet online. She began to dedicate twenty minutes each day to being mindful and appreciating her life, diseases and all. This, of course, did not mean she had to like her diseases. She didn't. But she did decide to accept them and not fight them. After she began meditating, Janice realized that for many years she felt that she was not enough. Even though she had been in and out of therapy her entire life, she still grappled with the history of having a father who did not participate in her life. Illness finally gave her a reason to look more deeply at her happiness level and dig deeper into why she always felt the world was against her.

> At first Janice thought her disease was just another bad card being dealt. But when she allowed herself to trust that perhaps her disease could be helpful to her belief that she was never enough, things started shifting and she was able to stop being so hard on herself. She was able to admire herself for doing such a great job in the midst of struggle. She stopped looking outside herself for validation of being enough like she wished her father had. Hashimoto's and celiac helped her stay on track to keep her focus on loving herself. She was able to find some appreciation for her circumstances. Janice changed her diet, started meditating daily, and began taking life day by day. She finally knew she was enough. And illness became her teacher to continually remind her.

The mindfulness notion may sound a little out there, or even difficult to believe, but we have science now that proves it to be true—that mindfulness, rest, and therefore love trigger a healing reaction in the brain and in the body, releasing positive energy. There is a somewhat scientific, albeit great, explanation that I'm simplifying a bit here from a *Scientific American* piece.[8] The brain has a fight-or-flight center. It's called the amygdala. It's the body's stress responder. A study by a researcher named Adrienne Taren of the University of Pittsburgh[9] did MRI scans that demonstrated that after eight weeks of practicing mindfulness, the amygdala shrunk. When the amygdala shrinks, the pre-frontal cortex becomes thicker. That's the part of the brain that helps you concentrate and make decisions. The testing also revealed that these two parts of the brain worked together to almost sharpen the brain's section that deals with concentration and attention. The more a patient meditated and practiced mindfulness, the greater the change in the brain. Disconnecting from the stress center in the brain through mindfulness seemed to increase both physical and mental health benefits. This study didn't suggest mindfulness was a cure-all for a terrible

---

8 http://blogs.scientificamerican.com/guest-blog/2014/06/12/what-does-mindfulness-meditation-do-to-your-brain/.

9 http://journals.plos.org/plosone/article?id=10.1371/journal.pone.0064574.

disease, but it did suggest a reduction of inflammation and stress markers like cortisol and interleukin, which are associated with some diseases.

In other words, mindfulness disconnects the stress department of your brain and in turn provides you with another tool in promoting good physical health. That means medicine alone or diet alone may not be the only tools to heal you. Meditation, love, and mindfulness, in conjunction with everything else, can help. A lot. At the very least, they can provide peace and calm that can lead to clarity or open the door for helpful and healing discoveries and happiness despite illness.

MOVING FROM MINDFULNESS TO APPRECIATION

Mindfulness seems to be evolving beyond just being mindful and into acknowledging gratitude and love for what is present. We know now that it actually affects the body. The emotion of appreciation can have a direct response in the body. But appreciation is a form of trust. It places our hearts and brains into a state of cooperation when we appreciate what is present—and it is quite easy to practice.

The Institute of HeartMath is a research organization that studies the connection between the heart and the mind. The organization's studies reveal that emotions don't come from the brain alone, but they also reside in the heart—that there's a link between the two, in fact, as they send information back and forth between each other. It makes sense, therefore, that emotions cause stress on the body. Do you ever feel exhausted after an ordeal? The body is responding to your emotions. Our heart beats faster when we're feeling anxiety or anger. The brain receives the message and then suddenly we can't think straight. It makes sense, therefore, that physical strain and illness are linked to mental strain.

But there's a flipside to HeartMath's research. The same interaction occurs with loving feelings. The messages move back and forth and create harmony in the mind and the heart. The brain feels good and the heart feels good, reducing the negative impact on our organs. Think about that: You can impact your heart by thinking loving thoughts, by generating warm emotions instead of negative ones. What a powerful message. You have healing power within you right now. You can positively influence your physical health and well-being. HeartMath reveals that feeling appreciation is a good way to generate positive emotions, which can then affect your physical body.

PRACTICE APPRECIATION

Here's what I'd like you to do right now: Generate some thoughts of appreciation. Write them down or just think about them—big or small.

What are you appreciative of? It can be something simple, such as the bus or train showed up on time. It can be something larger, such as my children are happy and well adjusted. Every day when you wake up, or when you're on your way to work, think of one thing that you truly appreciate. Even on your worst and most miserable days, there has to be something that generates appreciation inside of you. Even when you're struggling and can't see light at the end of the tunnel, think about what is good and positive in your world. Now recreate that feeling:

- What does it feel like to appreciate something good?
- Can you hold on to that feeling?
- Can you recall it when you're blue or struggling?

Don't think about an actual event or memory so much as the emotion surrounding it. That's the good stuff. That core emotion is what will boost you. Once you can generate these emotional triggers, great things will follow.[10]

When you learn to tap into these positive emotions, you will experience the following results:

---

10 www.rewireme.com/neuroscience/appreciative-heart-good-medicine/.

- Increase heart rhythm coherence
- Reduced emotional stress
- Improved health
- Stress reduction
- Increased emotional awareness
- Emotional balance
- Improved cardiovascular health
- Lowered blood sugar

Here's the bonus: Appreciation comes from within you. It comes from reflecting upon your own life and events in your life. Appreciation is a state of being. It doesn't require you to be anywhere other than where you are. And it's instantaneous. Appreciation for anything aligns you with the state of cooperation. And even more incredible, appreciation for what ails you can be powerful medicine. So an appreciation exercise is great because it keeps the work inside of you, it's multi-pronged, it changes your chemistry, and it keeps you in line with your own life and trusting that there may be some wisdom in your disease.

LOVE AND HEALTH

There's been much research lately that confirms the mind-heart connection, including this:

Study: Modulation of DNA Conformation by Heart-Focused Intention [11]

By Rollin McCraty, Ph.D., Mike Atkinson, and Dana Tomasino, B.A.

"During the experience of negative emotions, such as anger, frustration, or anxiety, heart rhythms become more erratic and disordered, indicating less synchronization in the reciprocal action that ensues

---

11 https://www.heartmath.org/articles-of-the-heart/personal-development/you-can-change-your-dna/.

between the parasympathetic and sympathetic branches of the autonomic nervous system.

In contrast, sustained positive emotions, such as appreciation, love, or compassion, are associated with highly ordered or coherent patterns in the heart rhythms, reflecting greater synchronization between the two branches of the autonomic nervous system."

The Loving Diet Translation: This means that the more kind and gentle we are for our circumstances, for our situation, and for our life, the easier our body operates. Science is in its first stages of making the connection that loving thoughts have the potential to heal. The bonus for you is that regardless of your diet, medications, and environment, you can start loving and potentially change your DNA with no side effects or dangerous interactions. Think of it as a free form of medicine available to you in unlimited supply.

CAN YOU CHANGE YOUR DNA?

What we're finding out is that when you're mindful, you're in a state of loving. When you're in prayer, mindfulness, meditation, or a loving state, it creates a biochemistry change in the body. It lights up different brain centers in the body, which encourages chemicals to be released from the brain, which promotes relaxation. Those are things that we know. Have you ever thought about what a miracle is? We've all heard of them—that person with stage 4 cancer who is spontaneously healed. How did that happen? Science hasn't proven it, but it's certainly being studied. I believe healing miracles are a manifestation of living love.

I believe healing miracles are a
manifestation
of living love.

💜

A MINDFUL MOMENT

For the next ten minutes, sit in a quiet space. Take some deep breaths
and center yourself. Think about something that makes you really
happy and use that feeling to fill up your body. Just sit with that feeling
for a moment. While staying in that moment, feel your happiness grow
bigger and expand in your body. See that happiness touch the places
in your body that may be in pain or affected by your disease. Imagine
your body completely whole just as it is. Spend a few minutes breathing
in that state of wholeness.

AFFIRMATIONS:
HOW TO FIND THE TIME

You brush your teeth, right? Take a shower? Then you have enough time
for an affirmation. Think about what you do while you brush your teeth.
Are you looking in the mirror at yourself? Thinking about who you have
to call or e-mail back? Replaying a bad conversation in your head? Great!
Then that means brushing your teeth is the perfect time for affirmations. Stand at the mirror twice a day, brush your teeth, and repeat your
affirmations. I keep affirmations on Post-it notes in my medicine cabi-
net—a perfect solution for anyone who thinks there is no time in the day
to say good things to yourself.

At the end of most chapters, I'm going to give you a few affirmations.
Say them aloud or in your head. Write them on Post-it notes and stick

them on your doors and cupboards. They work. At my darkest moments, I say them one hundred times a day. Some chapters will have exercises that will help you self-assess and will ultimately guide you to trust your life. These will help you be mindful.

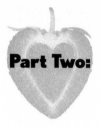

Part Two:

LOVE

We decide if our stumbling

blocks become stepping

stones.

4

LOVE YOUR STRUGGLE

Illness is grace in disguise.

💙

I WANT TO PRESCRIBE SOMETHING new to your health-care regimen, in addition to everything else you're doing to deal with your disease: *love.*

Love might help you heal. It's a free resource, so why not draw on it? It's unlimited. Plus, never has anyone in history ever said, "I want *less* love in my life." There's a bottomless pit and abundance of love, and most everyone wants more of it anyway. So why not use it? I'm not talking about the romantic relationship kind of love. I'm talking about something else completely. There are loving pieces in all of our lives that we can draw on. There's love everywhere. Drawing on love to heal is the crux of The Loving Diet. Once you see it and use it, happiness and joy will increase and you will create a healing environment, prompting physical healing to take place.

WHAT DOES LOVE LOOK LIKE?

Jennifer had been on the Autoimmune Paleo Diet for months. After being diagnosed with rheumatoid arthritis, she had heard about the diet from a friend. She dove in and dedicated herself to changing her diet and immediately felt better. She worked with her chiropractor and began taking some supplements that supported her overactive immune system. But after a few months of feeling better, she still did not feel great. So she decided to start *The Loving Diet* to create a more holistic plan for healing. Jennifer began starting her day by being open and willing to see rheumatoid arthritis as a tool of transformation. She did not know how it might transform her, but she was willing to wake up each day and trust that some kind of wisdom might be hidden within her diagnosis. She asked for more loving in her life every day. Every time she started to feel sorry for herself, and her joints began really aching, she would stop, take a deep breath, and say, "I trust my life."

Jennifer also visualized herself as whole, not broken. She loved herself more. She pictured herself complete, even though she sometimes felt like the disease was against her. When that happened, she focused on what a great job she was doing anyway. That was love. She started reflecting upon her marriage breaking up around the time her symptoms of RA began. She had often felt that she was in the way of her busy husband and his budding career. She felt like she always came second in the marriage, after his career. In her daily meditations, she started reframing her marriage. She had always wanted to teach art to children, and her husband never supported that decision. Maybe the rheumatoid arthritis and her marriage dissolving forced her to slow down for a reason? Maybe this disease could help her focus on her heart's true desire. Maybe her marriage was actually a distraction from her true calling—a calling that she never thought she was good enough to hear: being an artist who teaches others. Maybe life had been completely on track all this time. Beyond the heartbreak, beyond the life falling apart and the diagnosis of disease, life might actually be full of promise.

Jennifer was able to feel more peaceful about her divorce, her disease, and her circumstances. She enrolled in night classes to *obtain her teacher certification, something she would never have done while married. Her disease allowed her to take a different perspective. Life was not off track; it was actually on track. When she took the time to trust, examine, and reframe, the gifts became evident. Even though it did not change her diagnosis, it allowed her to be happy regardless. But in the process, she felt more connected to her body, and the pain lessened. She found a body worker who helped with the pain she was experiencing and finally discovered a new sense of freedom in her life. She was able to feel gratitude for how her life unfolded in the midst of struggle and pain, all thanks to love.*

STOP STRESSING ABOUT THE NOISE IN YOUR HEAD AND INSTEAD LOVE IT

My clients often tell me about how difficult it is to stop the negative thoughts that swirl in their heads. Sometimes, on certain days, it's really difficult to think of anything but the struggle. So instead of worrying about that noise, we should work to welcome the mire and the muck. After all, we're only human. There are days when we're going to be in it—that mire and muck. The more you can love yourself exactly where you are, the quicker you will get out of it. Believe it or not, if you can love that part of you that struggles with disease, then you naturally get into alignment inside yourself. You actually put yourself in a better position, because you're making an adjustment that aligns you with the loving.

That may sound complicated, but by loving everything and turning away from nothing—even the bad stuff like the struggle with your disease—your thoughts organically fix themselves. Love everything and stop avoiding the shadows of yourself. Love the pieces of you that aren't positive, because we all have them, they are part of us, and we're all just trying to get through it. Loving the bad in our lives ensures we turn lack into loving. That's how we then heal the quickest.

THREE THINGS I SAY TO MYSELF
WHEN I'M STRUGGLING

1. "I'm doing the best I can under difficult circumstances."
2. "This is hard right now, but this is temporary."
3. "Today is a pretty hard day to be a human, but things will get better."

STEPS TOWARD LOVING THE MIRE
AND THE MUCK

1. Practice self care.
2. Trust the timing of your life.
3. Know you're always on the right path.
4. Know that bad things happening doesn't equal a bad life.
5. Understand that suffering is part of being human.
6. You don't have to like your disease. Appreciate your life instead.

HOW TO LOVE

Love is the glue of the universe. It is the central theme of most major religions on the planet. So investing in love won't conflict with any religious beliefs you have. And it is possible to have the same feeling you have for someone you love, or a precious moment in your life, as you have for your illness and circumstances. It is simply a matter of allowing, choosing, and trusting. It may be normal to feel like if you love what ails you, you're giving it permission to be there, be the one in charge, and take over. This is a false belief. When you accept everything that contributes to your life, which is a loving action, you are investing in yourself. You are taking a perspective that uses everything in your life to lift you up, also a loving action. Acceptance may be the first step you take toward loving. Trust is also another step toward loving. The action of moving from against disease and the current state of your life is one of love. Even spending five minutes a day in acceptance of your circumstances can change how you feel about things.

EXERCISE ON ACCEPTANCE:

Waking Up to the Wisdom

Illness is trying to wake you up to something. Let's spend ten minutes exploring what that might be.

1. Sit in a quiet spot.
2. Close your eyes.
3. Take some deep breaths.
4. Imagine yourself, ten years into the future.
5. Imagine your future self walking into the room you're sitting in now meditating.
6. Look at your future self, and ask:
   - What wisdom am I supposed to learn?
   - How is this disease helping my life?
   - Will you give me some reassurance that I'm going to be okay?
   - What are the blessings of my disease?

Thank your future self for stopping by.

When you're ready, open your eyes.

From this, you'll learn that some day in the future, you're going to be in a different place in life than today. That might not mean healed, but when we experience crisis, it's important to know we'll be okay. It's nice to have someone tell you that you'll be okay. Your future self will be that person. Call your future self in any time you feel the need. All of this brings you into alignment, knowing you're on the perfect path for you—that ultimately illness is a resource for wisdom.

SUFFERING STILL EXISTS

Even with healing, suffering still occurs. When we decide that something is either good or bad, we've moved away from our center. You don't have to look at a really painful, horrible experience as a good thing. Who would, right? But maybe there was something else happening that you need to acknowledge. Even considering the notion that trust may be an option, and provide a benefit in some way, can help change biochemistry. Our mind and our ego want to compartmentalize everything and say *this is good, this is bad.* This type of thinking believes that the more good things you can add up in your life at the end, the more you win.

If you think like that, you're missing the point.

I'm asking you to move beyond that and above that. Let's look at the entire landscape of our life as being one event after another, propelling us toward fullness, because if we don't judge situations as good or bad, we can look at them as opportunities for wisdom, opportunities for choosing ourselves, opportunities for trusting our lives, and opportunities that something bigger is at play here, trying to help us find a deeper place of joy, abundance, and wisdom. That's love. Then, we can look at everything as simply one more step to getting there, and when we do that, it's not a stumbling block, it's a stepping stone.

If you can decide to make everything a stepping stone and not a stumbling block, then you attract stepping stones to your life instead of stumbling blocks.

No keeping score. No comparison and regret—both keep you from wisdom. Imagine you're in a hot air balloon and you are trusting how life is pushing you forward; it makes you go up even farther into the sky. Then, you're above the good and the bad. You're just looking at your life and, when you're doing that, you stop judging if something is *good or bad.* It doesn't mean that less bad things will happen to you, it doesn't mean that life will get easier; it means that you learn how to have a different perspective to keep re-orienting yourself every time something happens—that there's a benefit in there for you and your wisdom and your loving.

EXERCISE

How to Purge the Bad Thoughts and Replace Them with Love

Stop what you are doing right now and visualize your life on track. Visualize your disease bringing you closer to wholeness, not farther away. See what happens when you do. Do you feel a sense of peace? A sense of calm? Illness can be the constant friend, or a reminder to do this if you allow it. It is the allowing that is the secret sauce. Allowing, accepting, and appreciating are the three As of moving into a place of love. And after you start investing in the three As you can let go and see what comes forward.

In a sense, in choosing love, you become a seeker of the blessings in your life. No matter what life presents you with, you dedicate yourself to finding the gifts. And you can do this in the midst of struggle or pain. And doing so may even help the struggle and pain. So instead of bracing yourself against life's curveballs, you can start investing in the place inside yourself that will be all right in the midst of what life throws at you. There is tremendous freedom there because you're acknowledging that you can handle life from a loving place, not from a fighting place.

With illness, you're choosing to try to accept your life even in the midst of suffering. Doing so gives you a better shot at reducing that suffering. It's a tool to help you accept your life. It increases if you resist and don't accept your circumstances. Of course, we all encounter extremely sad things in our lives, such as loved ones dying. There's no way around that kind of suffering.

Ask yourself if you want to keep looking at life as though it is pushing you down, because life is never going to stop having hardships. The physical body is not built for perfection. Nothing in your life changes per se. You make a different decision about how you see your life. That's the part that changes.

Why not make it the *glass is half full* instead of the *glass is half empty*, which is another way of saying, *Is it a stepping stone or stumbling block?*

Then, you get to enjoy life and there are no mistakes. Everything becomes your training to be an ambassador of love toward yourself and your circumstances. You use everything that comes your way to your own benefit. It's as if there is no loss. You don't have to give up anything to take this perspective.

Allowing, accepting, and appreciating are

the three As of moving into a

place of love.

♥

A LOVING AFFIRMATION

Right now, I am already whole. I am not off track. Illness is here to draw me toward wholeness, not farther away. I am dedicated to finding the blessings in my life.

5

AVOID AGAINSTNESS

Choose not to identify yourself by your illness
but by your loving toward it.

💙

WE'LL TALK A LOT about againstness in the book—the notion of swimming upstream and fighting, inside and out. The very definition of autoimmune disease is tissue self-attack, which in itself—attack—is againstness. Againstness that is happening inside of the body. Spiritually, if we can remove the againstness everywhere else—in our minds and hearts as well as in our stomachs and bodies—then there will be a ripple effect toward the physical part of what we are struggling with. If we can find where someone is being attacked emotionally, flip and fix that by reframing it, then we create overall cooperation in the heart and, eventually, the body.

If you've tried endless treatments and seen multiple doctors, it's likely you're pretty beaten up about it all. Most people who come to see me are at the end of their ropes. Many have told me they've contemplated wanting to die because their illness has taken such a heavy toll on their lives. When I work with people, or when they attend a workshop of mine, by the end of it they find hope. They see light.

The first step is making you realize that your disease—Hashimoto's or MS or cancer—is not the enemy. Thinking your disease is the enemy is a limiting belief. Hating your disease creates againstness, which only creates more negativity in your heart, mind, and body.

WARDING OFF AGAINSTNESS

If something stressful and upsetting occurs in your life, such as getting diagnosed with an autoimmune disease, are you going to fight it or are you going to work with it? Most people opt to fight it. When faced with the news of an illness, most people react the same way. They receive the news from their doctor that the lab results revealed an illness, like multiple sclerosis, for example. First, they brace themselves in their mind, and then they go into shock. The second thing they do is almost universal. They say, "I'm going to fight it. I'm going to beat this illness. I'm stronger than this illness. I'm stronger than this." That reaction is very much standard across the board, whether someone gets cancer or heart disease or autoimmune disease. People immediately adopt warrior mode and proclaim they're going to change their diets, get healthier, work to mentally overcome the illness, and grow stronger for the long fight ahead. Most people vow to "beat the disease." We bolster ourselves in so many different ways, but fight is number one. We're told by society to not listen, because we're supposed to be fighting. We're expected to be strong. I'm suggesting taking the route of being vulnerable enough to consider that your disease could add to, not detract from, your life. Such a notion takes courage. That route asks that we believe in ourselves and be fearless for ourselves. That route asks us to use everything in our lives, including disease, to make it better.

There is a generally accepted perspective about disease in the United States: You have to be strong and you have to fight disease. If you want to overcome what is plaguing you in your life in the physical body, you have to get tough and you have to beat it. It's because society tells us that the people who are the strongest win.

I can understand why people approach an illness with that mentality, but I'm asking you to consider another line of thinking—something other than *fighting it* or *overcoming it*. Instead of saying to yourself that "something is wrong and I'm going to fix it," and therefore aligning yourself with what I call *againstness*, I'm asking you to love it. Love the disease. This won't happen overnight. But buy into the process that it might work, that it might be a resource. You might shift how you feel about your life and how you feel in your body.

I'm suggesting that a more rapid way to deal with your autoimmune disease is to love your way out of it, or love your way through it, or love your way into it. When *loving* is the action for the circumstances in your life, it instantly changes your biochemistry.

Instead of saying to yourself that "something is wrong and I'm going to fix it," and therefore aligning yourself with what I call againstness, I'm asking you to love it. Love the disease.

♥

AGAINSTNESS

When we produce againstness, we are not in cooperation with everything inside of ourselves. We have to go outside of ourselves to find answers when we align ourselves with againstness. Againstness produces an idea inside of our bodies, hearts, and biochemistry that suggests something is awry. Instead try the following:

- Eliminate the mentality that something is wrong and needs to be fixed.
- Resist the notion that you need to be on track and back on a specific path.

WHEN LIFE FALLS APART

Here's the deal: Life is going to fall apart in some way or some form, eventually. It is the human condition. You may get an autoimmune disease, lose your job, have your heart broken, or have someone you really love die. It simply isn't an option to be a human and come out unscathed. But you have a choice about how you want to react to your life falling apart. Are you going to trust it? And when it does, will you let love catch you? You get to decide what your relationship with the adversity in your life will be, and I highly suggest a cooperative one, since it gives you the highest likelihood of health, wealth, and abundance. It is the difference between trying to dig yourself out of a pit or sitting in the pit and decorating it with pretty things until the ladder is dropped down for you to climb out. It is our relationship to difficulty that ultimately provides the cure. It is not the doing or trying to change the difficulty that works.

MAKE IT AN OPPORTUNITY

I call just about everything that happens to us in a day an opportunity, even the bad experiences. We all have moments, for the most part, where life falls apart. When that happens, consider that what's really happening is that life is rearranging itself to come together in a better way. So that *life falling apart* is just a metaphor for something more powerful coming forward that can steer you in a new direction.

OPPORTUNITIES

The following situations can all offer opportunities for growth:

- Divorce
- Heartbreak
- A diagnosis of illness
- Failing
- Death

- Abuse
- Fertility issues
- Job loss
- Injury

We don't wish bad stuff upon anyone. It would be fantastic if life simply puttered along and never fell apart. But that's not the case. When these opportunities occur, your first thought might be that you simply can't make it through them. In fact, when life has borne down on me, often my initial reaction is "How the heck can I make it through this? I can barely get out of bed!" When painful situations occur, we often think that they're overwhelmingly terrible and they're going to leave our lives in ruins. On the surface, these situations may seem negative, but imagine if you could embrace and love them and learn that they might just mean that something better will come of them? There is some serious power in surrendering to the timing of your life in this regard. It can be painful and seemingly not make sense, but mostly you will be okay.

DON'T THINK POSITIVELY

When people say, "All will be okay if you just think positively," I want to stop and ask them, "Are you kidding?" We aren't built as humans to change the world at that level. That notion means you have to be a certain way, think a certain way, and eliminate sadness and negative thoughts. *The only way you have to be is the way you are right now.* I suggest a new consideration: Love the negative. Love the anger. Love the sadness. Love the panic attacks. Love the illness. Love the circumstances of your life. What do you have to lose by considering that option? The whole premise of The Loving Diet is that at your core you are whole, complete, and perfectly positioned for great happiness. That life sets us up for maximum learning by giving us experiences. Not all experiences are positive. In fact, positive thinking means you need to be somewhere else than where you're at. Positive thinking means you need to adopt something different in order to make your life better. The Loving Diet says that you're already whole and you're okay with who you are, and that it's okay to love the part of you that's sad. In fact, loving the sad you may be the quickest way out of being sad. And it's okay to love the part of you that's angry and scared. You are already okay even if life seems like it is not. You're just awakening to that. Positive thinking means you need to change something or do something to be positive.

FINDING RELIEF

Think about this: You don't need to do anything differently than what you're doing in your life. You are 100 percent the way you're supposed to be. Does thinking that give you a sense of relief? Does knowing that you're already there help you relax? You are right where you need to be. Knowing that can help you find the resources for healing disease. Consider there is a healing resource in the idea that you are on track for your life right now. By coming to that conclusion, you can change your health. You don't need to go anywhere to find the resources—you *are* the resource. A loving state creates a shift inside your body. And then the resources will come to you. A modernized version of the old term "As above, so below."

The ultimate timeless moment: knowing that wherever you're at you're okay. All the pieces are already there. You don't have to reach outside yourself for the wealth and the house and the love and the healing. When you're already whole, and you make that leap to loving all the pieces within you, then you don't have to go anywhere or do anything or be anything. You're already there. Illness is the teacher that's trying to teach you that you're already there.

BANISH THESE COMMON THOUGHTS FROM YOUR DIALOGUE

- Think positively.
- The healing is outside of you.
- There is a finish line—we've already crossed it by virtue of being born whole.
- You're off your path.
- There's a right way and a wrong way to do things.
- There's a formula for life.

EXERCISE:

Are You Living a Life of Againstness?

Answer the following questions:

- Do you often question the way your life is going?
- Do you feel a lot of opposition in your life with your relationships and work?
- Do you feel a lot of struggle?
- Do you often wish life were going in a different direction?

If you answered yes to most of these questions, you may have parts of your life in which you are producing againstness. Can you identify what is causing the againstness? The good news is that knowing there is againstness in your life in some cases is enough to help you move through it. Knowing it will loosen its grip. Now try to flush the againstness out with some affirmations.

A LOVING AFFIRMATION

I am willingly cooperating with my circumstances. I am taking full responsibility for my life. I appreciate the struggle in my life.

6

COME INTO COOPERATION
WITH YOUR ILLNESS

Be as radical in your forgiving as
you are in your loving.

♥

M ichelle was fifty and had struggled with Sjögren's and
Hashimoto's for much of her life. She used medication her
doctor prescribed for much of that time. Her naturopath told her
about the Autoimmune Paleo Diet and she went online to find out
more. She found The Loving Diet while searching for the AIP diet
and decided to try both. She immediately felt much better when
she eliminated grains, eggs, dairy, and nightshades. It took a
while to eliminate nuts and seeds, but eventually she was able to
get the hang of it. Michelle felt so much better that she was able
to work with her doctor and lower her medications. But still,
something was nagging her. She wanted to be happier and felt
like she worried a lot about how to manage her illness. She
wanted to go deeper into her illness and find out if there was more
to look at. She wanted to define her life by joy and happiness and
not by her disease.

Using The Loving Diet, Michelle started to reframe her ill-
nesses as an ally. She began imagining herself whole in the midst
of disease. When she started to feel worried about her disease,
instead of judging herself, she began to appreciate how her worry
had taken care of her. Her worry helped her find a new way to eat
and a new outlook on health. She soon began to realize that just

maybe her worry was not the enemy here. When Michelle started reframing her disease as being the constant reminder of her ability to take care of herself, she began to see patterns in her life that were not serving her. In the midst of doing this work, the memory of her parents' divorce when she was ten years old kept surfacing. She decided to pay attention to that memory. The more she thought about it, the more she realized that when her parents split, she felt responsible. She realized she decided way back then that she could not trust love. If her parents split, perhaps she would be doomed to the same fate? All decisions in her life from that moment on were made from that vantage point. But when she realized this belief she had formed (thanks to the illness that asked her to take a deeper look at everything), she realized she was deserving of trusting love and relationships. A eureka moment!

If Michelle had not had Sjögren's and Hashimoto's, she may not ever have realized that she was fully deserving of love, beauty, and abundance in her life. And in that moment, her life, even in the midst of disease, became the path she was walking all along. Her diseases were loving teachers helping her realize that life was guiding her to come to these conclusions, instead of moving her farther away from them. She could now wake up every day and see that she was not a victim of her circumstances; she was actually a finder of her own special blessings in the unfolding of her life. She never tried to push away the hard parts or remain positive after starting The Loving Diet. She used the hardest, saddest parts to take a closer examination of her limiting beliefs. And in doing that, she was set free. Her love and appreciation of her disease took her out of being a victim of her life. Joy became her loyal companion.

To be clear, none of this is easy. I don't want you to be reading this and thinking that for some reason I'm suggesting it's just a flip of a switch, and bam: love and trust. It's work. And sometimes it will take serious effort. For me it is a constant practice. Sometimes, you'll find the love and the trust and the ability to come into cooperation with your disease for one minute, and then you'll be right back in the gutter. That's okay. All of those one minutes will add up. They will all be beneficial. Eventually, the love and peace will extend to two minutes, then three, then an hour, and before you know it, you'll have come into cooperation with your illness.

THE DISEASE RABBIT HOLE

When we fall down the rabbit hole that can accompany disease, it sometimes feels like a cold, cruel descent. And during the entire fall down the hole, we are told some powerful messages:

- Reduce your stress.
- It's in your head.
- This medicine will help.
- Change your diet.
- Think positively.
- You don't look sick.
- Give it time; eventually you will feel better.
- Life is what you make it.
- Try this new medication.

I am sure you have a long list of things you have been told to do to manage your illness. And after years of these messages from a system that is not built to heal, after years of physical pain and suffering, my clients tell me they have come to the following conclusions:

- Joy died inside of me.
- I don't know how to be happy.
- I feel hopeless.
- This disease has robbed me of my life.

- Life is against me. The world is not safe.
- I don't know how to do this.
- Nothing helps.

And here is the kicker: Diet alone doesn't usually cure these conclusions you have made about your life. And neither does reducing your stress or eating nutrient-dense foods. Or taking B12 or getting a massage. The real-life issues of despair and loss of hope do not get solved with positive thinking. They get solved by being in a state of cooperation with your circumstances. You can follow a certain diet until the cows come home. And you may very well feel better. And your antibodies may drop. And your anemia may go away. But unless you examine the real root of what is trying to come forward in your life through illness, everything will be a temporary fix.

Illness is a vehicle that is trying to wake you up to something in your life. Illness is bringing forward the opportunity for finding, releasing, and healing the conclusions we have made about our life that are not serving us. Illness is the wisdom giver that teaches us that, ultimately, we find the road back to our own hearts by loving disease, not through being a victim of it. And so we get to do this. We get to sort through all the messages about how to get healthy. Some messages we hear out in the world are rooted in fear. Some are rooted in love. We use discernment inside ourselves, stemming from our yearning for more love, to decide what we align ourselves with. Because like a broken system so many of you know all too well, there also is a system with caregivers who operate from a loving place.

This is The Loving Diet. Putting the love back into our health care. Putting the love back into our diets. Putting the love back into our journey. Using disease as an opportunity to lift ourselves up. This is the path that changes the dark rabbit hole to a golden one. The route that goes beyond good and bad. Right now, ask yourself:

"How will I accept the loving?"

"What is preventing me from accepting the loving?"

But unless you examine the real root of
what is trying to come forward
in your life through illness, everything
will be a temporary fix. . . . Illness is
bringing forward the opportunity
for finding, releasing, and healing the
conclusions we have made about our life
that are not serving us.

FINDING COOPERATION

Americans generally see everything in black and white: Everything has to be positive and they don't allow any of the negative in. That's not an easy perspective to shake. We all feel it at times, some more than others. In the loving perspective, you're loving both sides of the coin. You're loving the part of you that's failing every day and messing up and tripping and stumbling. You're loving the sad and depressed person and the person who is sick and can't find the answers. And at the same time you're loving the person who has inside of her the ability to be a superstar, to choose wisely, to eat the healthy food, to be the social person, and to dress well and look put together. The loving piece is that you love both sides of the coin. You're not trying to run away from the hard part, from your shadow side. You're loving all of it. That's cooperation.

TAKING AWAY AN ILLNESS'S POWER

It might feel counterintuitive. But if you allow illness to work through you by loving it, then you're giving it permission to be there. You may feel that permission means you're okay with it staying there, and you may think, *Is this giving illness permission to kill me?* But that's not what I'm suggesting. If you give illness permission to come in, you're enabling it to give you some information—something you can learn or grow from—not to take over your life. It's sort of like the analogy of the big scary monster in the closet that gets bigger and scarier when you don't open the door, and your mind creates the worst scenario possible. When you open the door (a loving action), look at the illness monster, and give it a hug, you are actually taking away the power it has over you and establishing cooperation and love as the power. Then you can better understand what its role is in your life.

REASONS WE FEEL INCOMPLETE DUE TO ILLNESS

- Society tells us we are only a winner if we are healthy.
- We are taught that illness means something is broken.
- It is hard to feel complete when we are suffering physically.
- Illness usually sends the message that something is wrong.
- When we are sick, we feel as if we may have done something wrong.

A DIFFERENT KIND OF SYSTEM

You're working out of a different kind of system, one that has you thinking, *This illness is giving me some amazing information about how I want to re-examine my life. I want to explore my life from a deeper place inside myself that has the answers and knows that my worthiness is not based on how I look physically.* When we base worthiness on how we look physically, it's going to keep showing up. It's a physical thing, until we get it on a different level.

This is where people are, in some ways, more motivated, because when you think of autoimmune disease, which is not curable. It only can go into remission. It's like a hand up to your face all the time. It's there every single moment that you breathe. That's why when people are so sick of it, they're ready to try something different.

PERSPECTIVE

The more you come into cooperation with the illness itself, the more likely you're going to find something that's probably easier than you think it is. It could be a medication. It could be a practitioner. When you buy into this perspective of trust, believing that this illness could do something to benefit your life, then you can get really radical, and think, *I don't know how it's going to look, but I might be introduced to a practitioner who's going to understand exactly what's happening with my illness. She is going to be able to give me information I've never heard before that's going to change my perspective.*

When you bring the illness closer to you, you allow it to transform what's present. When that takes place, resources open up that you didn't know about before.

BY LETTING ILLNESS IN, YOU MIGHT:

- Come to a different, more useful conclusion about the role it has in your life
- Manifest a different kind of loving path for yourself
- Find joy in the midst of disease
- Find that it becomes less the focus of your life

MINDFULNESS IS A FORM OF LOVING AND COOPERATION

Mindfulness is just another version of cooperation. Loving is a version of cooperation. That means by being mindful, and therefore loving, we're cooperating with our life's circumstances—good or bad—whatever it presents us with. And loving, or being in cooperation with one's life, has an immediate impact. It works quickly. In an instant, loving changes biochemistry. It changes the parts of the brain that we use to process information. When we change biochemistry, we can change health more quickly. It's an internal process. You're not required to go out and do anything or go anywhere. It's a mindset that you choose in an instant, and it instantaneously changes the body. It's free.

For example, a woman named Alicia has numbness and tingling in her extremities. She can't walk quite right. She makes an appointment to see her doctor, as she should, and is diagnosed with multiple sclerosis, an autoimmune disease. Alicia can handle the MS diagnosis two ways.

Scenario Number One: The doctor might suggest medication, mostly to help prevent the disease from becoming worse. The medicine may or may not work, but that's what modern medicine offers. But Alicia does more than just take the medicine. She likely:

- Grieves and gets very upset
- Creates a plan to fight the illness
- Searches the Internet for "weapons" for her battle, including chat rooms, dietary suggestions, books, and support groups

Alicia is moving outside of herself to treat her illness. To be clear, The Loving Diet doesn't discount people taking medication or listening to a doctor's opinion. Instead, it offers a partnership.

Scenario Number Two: Alicia tackles her illness using The Loving Diet. She:

- Grieves and gets upset upon first hearing of her illness
- Wakes up the next day and decides that MS is going to be a teacher
- Decides that her life is not ruined
- Decides her life is not *off track*
- Understands and accepts that MS is not going to destroy her, even though she doesn't really know what the outcome of her health is going to be
- Cooperates with MS every single day
- Talks to MS
- Becomes friends with MS
- Actively works at not having any thoughts of trying to move out of the space that she's in, which is just the space of MS
- Does stress relaxation exercises
- Uses MS as a loving path

Simply deciding to approach her MS differently changes her biochemistry. That way, every day when she wakes up, she's open. She's creating openness to the idea that maybe other alternative methods will come to her.

She's open to all of the things that might come to her through being at peace with MS, or having the idea that MS is going to teach her something. It's more of an internal process of getting aligned inside of herself, knowing that some really wonderful things could happen here through her journey with MS. Next, the wonderful things are drawn to her. She might be attracted to a certain diet, or supplement, or a certain kind of practitioner. It's all an internal process, rather than struggling, againstness, fighting the MS, and reaching outside of herself and trying to find the answers. Instead, she's going on the inside and starting through the place of, *Everything is okay, even though I have MS. MS is here to teach me something. I'm going to learn something from it.*

YOU MIGHT NOT FEEL PHYSICALLY BETTER, BUT HAPPINESS CAN STILL BE AN OPTION

What I'm asking you to embark upon works, but it's not easy. In fact, it can be extremely difficult. I am asking you to come to terms with the fact that your disease can take you on different paths. You can get better. You can stay the same. You can get worse. Consider for a moment detaching from an expected outcome you might have (everyone wants to get better and I want you to get better, too, but when you trust your life and you take a loving path filled with appreciation for you circumstances, you let go of the outcome). Instead, focus on finding joy in the present moment, regardless of future outcomes.

Maybe you've already been through scenario one and fought and fought and fought. You're likely so frustrated and exhausted from fighting, but not improving, that you're looking for something that will help. Most of my clients are exactly where you are. They've taken warrior pose and vowed to beat their disease. It's fair to say you have to go through all of those things when you come into cooperation with illness. It's okay to be upset, angry, or sad. You just have to also buy into being okay with what's happening. You have to avoid againstness, which is what so many people do before seeing me.

Are you:

- Tired of fighting?
- Tired of not feeling better?
- Tired of seeing many doctors with some or little improvement?

Most likely you're also not happy. Autoimmune disease never leaves you. Once you're into the chronic stage where you're feeling pain or losing your hair, possibly daily, you've reached the point where you're willing to try anything to feel better. But love will help you feel like you have hope, regardless of your disease. It will help you feel like you're a human being again—a full and happy one. It will help you get clearer about what you want your healing to look like, and it will potentially help you achieve radical healing.

GETTING TO THE ROOT

I want you to take a moment to try to dissect what's at the heart of your issue and learn what in your past might be preventing you from coming into cooperation. First, ask your life: What is the problem? Next, ask the same question from a loving place. You have a genuine willingness in your life to see your disturbances as information toward wisdom.

YOU ARE ALREADY WHOLE

By birthright you are whole. Even with cancer or MS, we're all whole. If you can stop judging the disease and the diminished worth you feel you have experienced because of it, and the feeling that you won't be whole again until you're healed, you can find that wholeness. The judging takes us away from that idea of wholeness. It replaces it with the notion that we need to heal to be perfect. You're perfect regardless. That's what coming into cooperation with your circumstances will allow you to see.

When you love yourself, you aren't discounting any part of yourself when you do it. And from there, you'll get huge, radical magnificent healings. I believe we are all put on this planet to achieve our growth. All people are on their own path, the one that will provide them with the maximum amount of growth.

EXERCISE:

Meditation

Take fifteen minutes to complete this exercise. Sit quietly and take three deep breaths to center yourself. Imagine a gold light coming from the highest heaven into the top of your head. Have the intention of this gold light being pure love, here for your highest good. See this light gently roll into each part of your body, starting from the top of your head and slowly moving down your whole body. Feel it as warm, safe, and loving light. Almost like what liquid gold would look like. See it passing over all of the places in your body that are in pain, suffering, or diseased. Imagine this liquid gold transforming any diseased tissue, limiting thoughts or hurt emotions into healing teachers or allies that are working for you. Imagine those places gleaming with light, gold, and love. See your body transforming into a completely whole being from the gold light touching it.

- Notice if you feel any particular emotions when you do this. Do they have any messages for you?
- How are you feeling in your body when you do this exercise?
- Trust whatever surfaces. It might seem unrelated that a childhood experience might come to mind while doing this exercise. Trust that it's related and that it can help you.

This is a great meditation for anxiety and nervousness. I think it feels like getting cozy under a warm blanket. When you have let the gold light pass through your entire body, thank it for coming, take three deep breaths, and open your eyes.

A LOVING AFFIRMATION

I can do this. The universe never gives me more than I can handle. I get the choice every moment to use my challenges to improve my life. Everything coming present in my life is here to help me gain wisdom.

7

REDEFINE HAPPINESS

Illness has the potential
to bring you closer to wholeness,
not farther away from it.

♥

*M*imi was a stay-at-home mother with three children under the age of ten. She was diagnosed with multiple sclerosis (MS) a few months after her third child was born. She was terrified MS would eventually prevent her from taking care of her children. Immediately after being diagnosed, she sought out an alternative medical practitioner. She found a chiropractic neurologist who started her on a regimen of anti-inflammatory supplements and took a very close look at her blood chemistry. Together they discovered she was anemic and had insulin resistant hypoglycemia and SIBO. It was also suggested that she adopt the Autoimmune Paleo Diet, in addition to tackling those other issues her regular doctor had missed.

After searching the Autoimmune Paleo Diet online upon her chiropractor's suggestion, Mimi found The Loving Diet and my version of the AIP diet. We had a consultation, and she immediately got started. It was really difficult at first. She had horrible brain fog, anxiety, and was constantly hungry. But she kept at it. After a few weeks, she had a dramatic decrease in her brain fog and she could walk without a cane. The numbness and tingling in her left arm went away. She was so excited to be seeing results that she found confidence to keep following the diet, even though it was taking a lot of her time to prepare food and be a stay-at-home mom.

Mimi began thinking about when the symptoms (which she ignored for years out of fear) of her MS first started. It was in college. Sad to leave home, she moved three hours away to her new school. She found it hard to make friends and noticed she started to get stomachaches quite regularly. She struggled in school and spent a lot of time feeling sad. She missed her family and friends at home. Looking back, it seemed odd that there might be a connection to this time, but she trusted that this nugget of wisdom appeared so that she would look at the time she started not feeling well. Once she embraced The Loving Diet, she began doing visualizations and meditations, focusing in on that college time to see if anything surfaced. She woke up every morning and looked at the affirmations around her house:

- I trust my life.
- I intend to use MS as a teacher for more wisdom in my life.
- I am actively seeking the blessings from this disease.

Each day after everyone went to bed, Mimi would sit for fifteen minutes (it was all she had time for with three kids) with her journal and talk to her MS. She started asking it very pointed questions like, "MS, is there a link to you and how sad I was when I went away to college?" or "MS, I would like you to tell me what gifts you are going to offer my life." She had no expectations when sitting. In fact, she focused mostly on how proud of herself she was for maintaining the diet and setting aside fifteen minutes during her jam-packed days! Eventually, the MS started to speak to her.

One day during her quiet time, she had a flash that life was turning into a disappointment, and that it had all started when her college experience was so difficult. Mimi thought about this for a while and began to see all the places this belief was woven into *her life. Lovers who had left, jobs she had lost, her health "giving up on her" when she got MS. All of it was really hard. She was sad about this realization for days. She allowed herself to feel sad that life was letting her down. She gave herself permission to be sad for as long as she needed to, and at the same time, she actively believed there may be some kind of wisdom in uncovering this belief she had. She forgave herself for believing that life was not showing up in the way she expected. Then something different started happening. Mimi began waking up happier. When she gave herself permission to feel sad that life was not going the way she dreamed it would, she stopped holding onto the expectations of how it should look. She started to change the picture in her mind of a successful life. She began to accept her MS diagnosis and not hate it as much. After all, it was the MS diagnosis that forced her to look deeply at her life and find a way to be happier. Mimi started to accept that she did not know the outcome of her disease, but that right now, at this moment, life was going to work better for her because she was letting go of her expectations.*

Mimi realized that in college her expectations were quite high. She expected things to be so easy. But, looking back, she developed some really valuable skills in college she had not noticed before. She became a much more compassionate person. She learned how to do things by herself. She faced her shyness by joining some on-campus clubs. Maybe she had not been so far off the path after all? Each time Mimi sat at night, she started to imagine her body whole and to have friendlier thoughts toward her MS. She started to see that perhaps MS could be a resource for her. And when she felt an MS flare starting, she got scared, yes. But she stopped feeling rage and hatred toward her body. She used it as signal that her body had something important to tell her. She became a very wise listener to her body. And each time that happened, Mimi felt a sense of relief that she had the tools to use everything in her life to help her, instead of feeling like she was being attacked or was a victim of her disease.

ARE YOU HAPPY?

Take this happiness quiz. Ask yourself these questions and write down the answers in a journal.

1. What does happiness feel like to you?
2. Where do you think happiness comes from?
3. Do you think it's possible to simultaneously have a disease and be happy?
4. Do you feel confident that life is unfolding for your benefit?
5. Do you feel happiness in the midst of suffering?
6. Do you feel purpose on your life's journey?

As you answer these questions, review how life has unfolded for you. Do you see your experiences as opportunity? Think of it like a video game. When a hurdle or struggle comes at you, how quickly can you come into cooperation with it? Then you suffer less. Don't disregard the pain; pull it closer. Trust that it's the best thing for your life. My therapist calls this the soul-fire-burn, seeking God more quickly. You go down super deep, but you go down super deep trusting your life. Happiness for me comes almost 100 percent from trusting. When I live in trust, all I have to do is reformulate situations and experience them as a human. I don't have to do much else.

THE HAPPINESS FACTOR

What is happiness? When you have an ailment, being happy doesn't mean you have to be happy all the time. Health, wealth, abundance, or joy can exist alongside or alternating between physical pain and struggle. It's accepting that it's okay to feel the struggle while you're struggling, and that alone is a form of joy—that you're okay even though you're depressed.

Happiness is getting to the place where you realize:

- My life is okay.
- I'm okay.
- I'm worthy of love.
- Loving can come to me.
- I can have an abundant life and still have a chronic disease.

That's really the goal. That's happiness in a sense. When you can buy into that idea, that you're still okay and you're not fighting the sadness, you're not fighting the anger, and you're not hiding, but rather you're letting all of the sadness and the anger come along with it, then you're still loving yourself while that's happening. That's happiness.

> Happiness is getting to the place where you realize: I can have an abundant life and still have a chronic disease.

APPRECIATE THE STRUGGLE

Suffering comes from not being okay with what is present. Every day, we wake up, we look at our lives, and we aren't okay with something. So we struggle against it because we want it to be different. For some people, the struggle is:

- I don't want cancer.
- I don't want MS.
- I don't want Hashimoto's.
- If this man loved me, then my life would be okay.
- If I had more money, everything would be great.
- My job is horrible.

We are constantly trying to change how life is. The opposite side of that coin would be:

- Everything is in alignment.
- The timing is perfect in my life.
- This is the way it's supposed to be.
- All my relationships are teaching me things about myself.
- I get to decide how I feel about my life.
- I am a student to all my experiences.

When you appreciate the struggle, then you're moving into cooperation with what's present. That's a one-way road to enjoying your life. Difficult and a stream of continual work—all the time essentially—but worth it to find that joy.

Most of you reading this are suffering with an illness, but heartbreak is one of the best tools we can use to understand what I'm trying to teach you here. We always want heartbreak to look differently. We wake up in the morning, facing a break-up or demise of a marriage, and we wish it looked another way or played out differently, and think to ourselves that if it had, then we'd just be happy.

On your next bad day, instead of wishing it to be different, take a couple of deep breaths, see it as it is, and know:

- Everything is okay.
- It's the way it is supposed to be.
- Nothing is out of sync.
- You're on schedule.
- Even though this is happening, you are okay.

You'll find that eventually you're able to reassure yourself and feel better about yourself.

EXERCISE:

What Are You Struggling with Right Now?

- Think about the person, place, or thing you are struggling with.
- Sit for a moment and picture it or them in your mind.
- Let your feelings toward it/them surface.
- It is okay if you can't stand them or the situation. (Most likely scenario, actually.)
- Ask the Divine to show you the way out of this.
- Say it in your mind a few times. It could be: "God show me what to do" or "Divine, please give me some useful information right now."
- Then, picture them or the situation with a little golden box.
- Allow your mind to blur out the person or situation if you want to, but focus on the box. Intend for the box to have instructions or information inside of it for you.
- Walk over to the box and open it. See what it says to you. It could be a piece of paper with some note or it could be a verbal message.
- See if anything appears.
- I continually ask for guidance in my life. Every day, in fact. I ask you to do the same.

EXERCISE:

Seven Things You Can Say to Yourself to Appreciate the Struggle

1. I am doing a great job struggling.
2. The universe is supporting me in every moment.
3. This, too, shall pass.
4. I accept and love myself.
5. I trust that this struggle has a message of wisdom for me.
6. Everything is going to be okay.
7. It is okay to feel scared right now. I know I will get through this.

DISRUPTION CAN CREATE AN OPPORTUNITY FOR JOY

If someone receives a diagnosis of lupus, she might feel as if her life has been turned upside down—like everything that was normal has suddenly been disrupted. That's a fact. My client Bree felt this way when she was twenty-five. Bree had always considered herself to have a beautiful life. She was an aspiring model and college graduate. She came to me to change her diet and her outlook, after receiving some difficult news about her health. She was in a massive grief state after being diagnosed and understandably upset. But I asked her (like I am asking you) to imagine that there was a realm of possibility where that diagnosis comes forward for a person and inspires her to make a different decision about her life. Maybe she pursued something new to study, maybe after much reflection she learned that she was worthy of love and loving relationships, which prior to lupus she had not felt. It was the disruption of the disease—that shake in the foundation—that took someone from her daily routine to a new perspective and provided her with a moment to come forward and get down to the bottom of a situation, resolving something for her. That's when disruption can seemingly unwind itself in a beneficial way.

Bree had to completely overhaul the direction of her life. She no longer had the stamina for full-time modeling. As we dove into what that meant for her, it turned out she felt immense pressure to be pretty, growing up in a family that placed high importance on looks and charm. Considering walking away from modeling, she found herself in a place of pain and bitterness. Once she gave herself permission to be angry and bitter, she cycled through it quite fast and started tapping into the real emotion of her lupus: sadness and fear of failure. In some respects, her family's worst nightmare came true. Their beautiful model daughter had tragedy strike her life. Or did she? She came to The Loving Diet and changed the way she ate and immediately felt better. She also found out that she was gluten intolerant.

Bree dove headfirst into her new diet and began to sort through the sadness that had come forward with her lupus diagnosis. She never felt pretty enough or good enough, even though she was a model. Her romantic relationships never seemed to work out, because she always chose men that liked her for her looks and not for her heart. But when she started embracing the sadness of her lupus and her disrupted career, she realized that there was an unknown gift coming to her. It turned out that Bree had always loved health, food, and nutrition. But she always felt afraid to let her passion lead her life because everyone in her family was a high achiever and perfect looking. Now, by turning the disruption into something else, Bree learned she could help others with lupus and study nutrition. She became a nutritionist and found herself thriving in the middle of her dream job, helping others find hope in the midst of struggle. If lupus had not come forward and touched her life, she may never have examined what would really make her happy.

And because she took the time to embrace all of the emotions surrounding her diagnosis, Bree was able to live in a more authentic place for herself, accepting all the parts of her soul, not just the most attractive ones. She also found a relationship based on mutual love and respect. It was when she gave herself the love and respect on the inside to live the life that felt best to her that she received it on the outside with her relationship. Lupus was the teacher. Bree was the student.

UNRAVELING CAN LEAD TO DEEPER HAPPINESS

Disruption can be the universe's way of unraveling what we think is true, so that something more truthful can come forward into our life like in Bree's case, which can lead to a more genuine type of happiness.

It's different for everyone. For some people, disruption can resolve old trauma, eliminating a negative space and leaving them feeling lighter. For other people, it can resolve beliefs that held them back and prevented them from feeling fully happy. All of these require pure willingness. For some people, it can be about drawing their wealth and their health and their happiness from a heart-centered state, not from a materialistic or a physical state.

An illness enables us to move beyond the physical into the deeper aspect of where we derive our resources. That's the part about trusting your life and the disruption that's entered into it. When I got my heart broken into a million pieces by my husband, and we eventually divorced, I decided to transform my heartbreak by investing more fully in my own life and trusting others. It's pretty scary to be vulnerable now in a relationship, but the disruption of heartbreak is helping me to gain more loving in my life. And it doesn't mean I won't get my heart broken again. But it does mean that when I do, I have a different framework to operate from that holds me better. For me, the disruption caused by heartbreak unraveled some beliefs I had about myself, which was that I actually am deserving of loving, that I am worthy of having a loving life. That I can depend on life, that the world is safe, that God hasn't forgotten about me. Even in the midst of more heartbreak, I can hold those things to be true now. And you can as well in the midst of disease. Those core issues that I worked out through heartbreak (deserving love, worthy of a loving life, and the world is safe) are examples of core issues that people can work out through disruption to discover the happiness that stems from trusting your life and embracing love. Even though mine came through heartache, you may have similar issues that you resolve through disease. Everyone's path on the planet is unique, but safety, security, and loving are important resources in finding true happiness.

TALK TO THE BLOB

How do you find joy in the middle of a disease? Or a crippling accident? Or a painful loss like a divorce, death, or layoff? We can call it autoimmune disease, heartbreak, or natural disaster, but I call it *Joy in Disguise*. From disruption emerges joy.

Because what is joy after all? My definition of joy is "the propensity of something to cause an upliftment in your life." And disease is no exception to that definition.

Try the following exercise:

- Take a few breaths and close your eyes for a minute.
- When you feel centered, ask your mind to let go of any definitions of good or bad for just a minute. That means you let go of the idea that disease is bad.
- For that minute try to see your disease as neutral. It is not destroying you; it is not healing you; it is merely a benign blob in the corner of the room.
- Now, I want you to look at the blob and ask it very seriously what gifts it plans to give you. It may be a staring contest, but smile and be patient while you hold your turf and see what it has to say.
- If it gets snarky and says "None," tell it that you love it. Tell it you love it so much that you have the patience to sit and wait for thirty more seconds for it to give you an answer. See what happens.

This is a great daily practice to remove the power you think disease holds over you and start redefining the relationship you have with it. It is an exercise of truly making peace with your difficulty. The exercise accomplishes two things: First, it allows the mind to stop promoting the idea that your disease is something "bad" or a major thorn in your side; second, it allows you to open yourself to the idea that your disease is an ally that is *on* your side, promoting the best for you—like the woman with MS, who used it to write a book and change thousands of lives. Or the woman with fibromyalgia, who finally got out of an unhealthy marriage. Or the celiac mother, who used her knowledge to catch the same disease in her child and applied it to help heal his autism. It goes on and on and on, and I believe it is simply a matter of finding the golden thread in your experience and pulling it to unravel its beauty and the joy it holds for you. I have seen what happens when people find their golden thread and pull on it. Beauty comes forward. Healing comes forward. Acceptance comes forward. Happiness comes forward. *You* come forward.

So I invite you to talk to the blob in the corner. I encourage you to consider just for a moment that you have been given the gift of *joy in disguise* and the messenger has been autoimmune disease.

People see disruption as a bad thing. Our mind speaks to us in a negative self-talk when destruction occurs: "Oh, look, life is against me. I'm having a disruption." Reframe that statement: "Oh, look, life must have something important to tell me because I am having a disruption." That's what I want people to do. Once they tweak their perspective, they will see that disruption isn't a "bad" thing anymore. Disruption is that wisdom coming forward, pushing us to trust life so that we can figure out what it has to teach us for our own greater happiness.

Political disruption changes systems. The independence of the United States occurred out of disruption. Positive change follows disruption if you choose for it to do so. Here's the key: If you decide to not take responsibility for your life and to remain a victim, then a victim is what you're going to feel like. The key is that you have to trust it and you have to choose it. If you don't trust illness and you don't choose the intention of finding out the wisdom coming forward from it, then it's not going to take place. Finding happiness within your experience of living with autoimmune disease is possible when you recognize the deeper growth and change that can occur within you. No one—or no particular set of circumstances—can bring you real, lasting internal happiness. Only you can make yourself happy—through your choices, perspective, and trusting your life.

A LOVING AFFIRMATION

Everything I experience in my life is here to help me in some way. I am willing to take a loving perspective toward my life. Happiness is an inside job and I'm up for it.

8

DON'T BE A VICTIM

Your relationship
with your illness matters.

♥

WHAT DOES BEING A victim look like? At its simplest form, it is anything besides taking 100 percent responsibility for your life or circumstances. That means any time you blame anyone for anything, you place yourself in the role of victim. And believe me, I have tried every which way to wiggle out of this definition. When my husband left me, I spent a good long while being a victim and feeling sorry for myself. I wanted all of my friends to take my side and feel sympathy for me. Why? I felt better when they did. It made it easier. I had less work to do when I could blame others for my fate. And every time I did this, I circumnavigated the wisdom of my struggle away from myself. I shortchanged my loving. Eventually I learned not to do this and I was the sole promoter of my circumstances, but it took a good long while to stop associating my self-worth with my experiences. Instead I learned to define myself by my loving my circumstances, as I ask my clients to do in The Loving Diet.

When something goes wrong in our lives, we immediately try out the victim mentality, aligning ourselves with the victim both inside and outside of our system. We almost try it out automatically, to see if it works. Once we do that, it cements us. And then it spirals. The victim perspective attracts victims. The fact is: It's much easier to blame someone else. It's easier than taking responsibility, because nothing is your fault. It's not easy to look inside yourself and see what you allowed to happen.

Instead of taking the victim route with your illness, claim it. Claim your mess. Claim the good. Claim the bad. Take 100 percent responsibility for your life. Doing so moves you out of the victim role and into loving and cooperation. That can happen organically if you claim everything—not only the good, but everything that makes up your life.

SIGNS YOU'RE BEING A VICTIM

The following three behaviors are a clear indication of a victim mentality:

- You blame anyone other than yourself: doctors, the world, God.
- You identify yourself with your circumstances instead of your loving toward it.
- You do not take 100 percent responsibility for your life.

This doesn't mean illness is your fault. It's more nuanced than that. Knowing you haven't created it is different. We don't willingly create disease. But if, for a moment, we could take the perspective that disease could be here for a purpose to help us uncover wisdom, happiness, and truth about who we are, perhaps it may seem less like the enemy. Plus, being proactive in addressing it and owning it skips the victim stage. When you're doing everything you can, bringing the love into your life, then you're not blaming someone else. There's a difference between blaming and accepting. Accepting is a position of cooperation, and cooperation for your life is a state of trust and love. And that is the place where healing can begin.

ESCAPE THE VICTIM MENTALITY

Take the following steps to avoid thinking of yourself as a victim:

- First, decide that you're going to take 100 percent responsibility for your life and your circumstances.
- Then keep the process going—it's constant.
- Remind yourself regularly by giving yourself permission to take responsibility so you don't fall back into a victim mentality.
- Keep choosing wholeness.

You'll experience an instant change simply by deciding to move away from the victim role. It's an instantaneous shift. You will feel more empowered, because you are choosing to trust your life. You might waffle in and out of being a victim of your life's circumstances, but even if you spend thirty seconds in that state of cooperation with the present and taking responsibility, that changes the moment. Even thirty seconds of acceptance allows the cooperation to come in. And when you allow cooperation to come in, you align yourself with cooperation, and life shifts in that moment. Many of my clients, once they have shed the victim mentality, have felt better. They have felt joy and happiness, and eventually their bodies start to feel better and even calmer. Ideally, you will want to spend twenty-five minutes day in the state of cooperation. Mindfulness studies confirm that this is the amount of time we need to spend daily on investing in cooperation to hardwire changes in our brain.

Many of my clients, once they have shed
the victim mentality, have felt better.
They have felt joy and happiness, and
eventually their bodies start to feel better
and even calmer.

♥

EXERCISE:

How to Stop Being a Victim

1. Decide you don't want to be one.
2. Accept all the parts of yourself that may be resistant to that. We want to keep up appearances and seem strong to others, so it may be hard to admit when we are being a victim.
3. Work with a therapist to help flush out unrecognizable victim behavior. It can often be subtle.
4. Look at all the places in your life where you don't want to accept responsibility. Make a list. Perhaps, how much you hate your job? Or are feeling stuck in a relationship? Or are feeling you have no choice about healing your body?

A LOVING AFFIRMATION

I trust my life. I take full responsibility for my life. I love myself even though I am sick. I have compassion for myself for choosing to be a victim. It seemed the easiest way! But now I am fully in charge of my life.

9

TRUST YOUR LIFE

Adversity is your opportunity.

♥

USED TO BE THE person with OCD tendencies. I said the Lord's Prayer ten times when I boarded a plane, and if I did not do it before the plane departed, I was convinced it would crash. I did not go anywhere without hand sanitizer. I would call moms up before play dates and make sure no kids were sick before dropping off my daughter. I was a huge worrier.

Maybe you can relate to this: Because we're human beings living in this physical world, we think we know what it should be like. Part of trusting life is that you have to trust however it's showing up. In some ways I feel like that's enlightenment. When you can live life fully in that state, that's yogi status. Yes, it's like the person who is going down in a plane crash and saying, "This is how it was supposed to be. Today I'm supposed to die in a plane crash," which you can do, because I'm almost to that place now where that's how much I trust my life. But again, it doesn't mean I don't suffer or hurt or ache. I absolutely do! It means that when I do, I trust it. There is something bigger in my life purposing that event that has my best interests in mind: growth and wisdom.

START BY SHOWING UP

When you consider the idea that you can trust illness, heartache, and life as you know it falling apart, you are buying into a powerful belief. You are buying into evolving toward wisdom and love. For me, trusting my life was accepting the idea that I can and should relinquish control in my life. That I should stop trying to control the direction of my life all the time. In essence, it is akin to taking your hand off the steering wheel of life. When you do, you invest in the idea that everything in your life is propelling you toward wholeness. In most cases, I don't know what that is. I can't say for sure. For me personally, it tends to be lessons about trusting myself and having faith in my own loving. For others, it is about safety and security. It's almost like a Buddhist way of life when you start meditating and you enter that space of stillness and trust. What is the stillness anyway? We don't really know and science hasn't really proven that. But what we do know is that paying attention, or mindfulness, can change how the body responds to stress, how it manages illness, and how the brain responds to stress. And that in itself could be a reason to invest beyond diet, supplements, and medication.

What I see with my clients, anecdotally and toward me, is that when you buy into not having to try as hard and simply show up, happiness, abundance, wealth, and health appear in a different way. Mindfulness succeeds when you aren't trying so hard but are instead trusting what is. Yes. For everything in my life, I do this. For me, it extends beyond health. I practice it in all aspects of life. It seems counterintuitive to do less in your life, but in some way this is what I am suggesting. Or rather, go ahead and keep trying, but attempt to control less. I always think about that old trick and metaphor: Throw the spaghetti noodle against the wall and see what sticks. I definitely try to work hard in my life, but I am less concerned with the outcome now. I do as much as I can and then I focus on letting go and trusting what materializes. I do this for my life, my health, and my relationships. What is the upside to this? I worry less, I trust more, and I enjoy life much, much more, because I cleared out so much space once occupied by worrying about the outcome, which I can now fill with joy.

TAKE SMALL STEPS TOWARD TRUST

Trusting my life was a process. I was resistant to it at first because I feared in doing so I had the potential to lose my mind. I found it uncomfortable to trust my life, but I managed my fear by taking it a little at a time, instead of diving in completely. I learned that it was not an overnight event, but rather I dipped my toe in the water to test it, bit by bit. And guess what? I still practice this. Because life does not stop throwing curveballs (read: I have more wisdom to awaken to), I still practice questioning everything and reinvesting in trust. As I write this, I am once again nursing a broken heart. Still, I struggle to follow my own advice. My cycle, and I'm certain you'll recognize this, looks something like this:

- I feel sadness and pain.
- I question my choices.
- I try to get out of horrible suffering.
- I consider options to numb my pain.
- I try out victim for a few days.
- I feel immense regret for letting myself be vulnerable.

But I turn things around eventually, and that's what I want for you, too. When I do, it looks something like this:

- Eventually, I sink back into the trust, the wisdom, and the bigger lessons at play.
- I give myself full permission to feel the uncomfortable waves of grief.
- I still continue to follow my own example and do this work daily.

- Each time I get dealt a curveball, I know what to do.
- I have the skills now to widen the wisdom and broaden my heart.
- Some days it is easy. Some days it is hard.
- On the hard days, I am extra gentle on myself.
- On the easy days, I congratulate myself.

TRUST YOUR EMOTIONS

*R*ose called me because she was suffering from horrible hives. *She had been to a dermatologist and her internist. She had followed their directions to take steroids and the hives came back. She went to an allergist and took an allergy test with no positive results. I suggested she get her thyroid tested, since hives can be associated with Hashimoto's. It turned out she was producing thyroid antibodies. But her doctor refused to help in any way because he did not think she was sick enough.*

We walked back in her life and looked at all the triggers that might have brought this on. Rose had recently readied her house for sale and painted her entire home. That was when her hives began appearing. When she made the connection that toxins from paint exposure could be the culprit of her issue, she felt a huge sense of relief. Rose started the Autoimmune Paleo Diet and began taking some thyroid-regulating supplements her chiropractor had recommended. She immediately felt better.

When we started talking about moving and the change moving can bring, she was immediately brought to tears. It turned out Rose was afraid of moving, and uprooting her sons from their school, so her husband could relocate for a new job. She was scared to leave her supportive community and try a new place to live. It made sense that she would question moving and felt sad. She had a belief that if she allowed herself to feel sad, she would not be supporting her husband. When Rose forgave herself for believing she was not important, she resolved her difficulty surrounding the move. She was able to let herself experience all the normal emotions of sadness and letting go of her home, while trying to re-establish herself in a new place. Her stress dramatically decreased when she made the connection that her health issues were leading her on to something: It is okay to take care of yourself. In fact, it is vital.

EXERCISE:

Consider the Idea

This may sound challenging, but take as an example a Hashimoto's diagnosis. Perhaps it's here to help you, not harm you. Just consider that for a moment. Today, I want you to think about your ailment and simply consider the notion that it's a positive. You don't have to figure out exactly what that positive is at the moment, just that something good may come from your disease. Don't do anything else, nothing drastic, just ponder that thought today.

THE GOAL OF TRUSTING YOUR LIFE

Simply stated, I want you to get more joy out of your life. You may not get better physically, but you will feel some measure of happiness in your life. Maybe that happiness leads to healing. The essence of trusting your life is believing that whatever is present in your life is here for your soul's growth. Once you do that, you won't have to worry about anything else. For me, I no longer spend energy worrying about all sorts of things, because I have a deep trust that everything that is here now is as it should be. Taking that perspective means I don't have to control things like I used to, which frees up space for happiness. Everything I might have worried about before is here to teach me something.

Now, instead of worrying, I focus on discovering what the struggle is here to teach me.

The essence of trusting your life is
believing that whatever is present in your
life is here for your soul's growth.

♥

EXERCISE: I

Trust My Life

Tomorrow when you wake up, I want you to do one simple thing. I want you to say, "I trust my life." I do, multiple times a day. When times get tough, say it more often. When I was going through my breakup with my husband, sometimes I would repeat this mantra one hundred times a day. Don't get me wrong—I didn't ever believe it at first. Not at all. But I was so motivated to find a way to feel better and find happiness and work through my sadness, that I just kept reciting it. Eventually, I actually believed it and the worry and stress of all that I hadn't trusted before evaporated.

TRUSTING YOUR GRIEF = TRUSTING YOUR LIFE

I had no choice but to eventually trust my life. The truth: Nothing else was working for me. When my husband and I broke up, the grief and pain were so horrible that nothing I did, except for sleeping, alleviated it.

Trusting your life is a perspective. With illness or struggle, you have to trust the grief. Grief is concentrated sadness. When people are in the grief state, life can seem unbearable. I remember thinking, *I totally know why people do drugs.* I felt that deep despair of wanting to numb all of my feelings. I knew instinctively at my low why so many people turned to alcohol or drugs to dampen the pain. That wasn't an option for me. I wanted to make an effort to ease my suffering. At the time, I was working with a woman who does energy work, and she said, "Have you ever thought about loving the grief?" My response: "That's the most ass-backward thing I have ever heard. That is not going to help."

But since I was suffering so intensely, I thought about it. My clients are sort of at the same stage. A doctor may have already told them that she has done everything possible and that she's out of solutions, or she's out of ideas. It's that sort of despair that makes people open and willing to hear another idea.

What does loving grief look like with disease?

- MS can give me the life that I want.
- My life can be better.
- I can get the life that I want through the midst of heartbreak.
- I can get the life that I want through a cancer diagnosis.
- Disease can be a teacher and a powerful tool.

It's safe to trust your life, by taking the perspective that illness is a powerful ally, here to teach you something that will benefit you. Here's another way to look at it: When you consider success in America, people are pretty rigid about how they define achievement. Success in this country is based on black and white, good and bad. When your friend gets diagnosed with breast cancer then something is wrong with her life—it's seen as the opposite of success and it takes away the possibility that her life can still be a success. We all say, "Oh, look at what just happened to her. Breast cancer ruined her life." My perspective is that every event in our lives—even the cancer diagnosis—is here to help us to become more whole. Becoming more whole is becoming more loving. Being born on this planet gives you that right. Disease means we're off mark to most. Trusting that it's part of your life, and only one aspect, means it's not off mark, it's okay. I'm asking people to see beyond the traditional measure of success and know that everything that makes up our life, both the good and the bad, is what actually makes us whole.

DISTORTED MEASURE OF SUCCESS IN AMERICA

Most Americans perceive success in the following ways:

- If you have money, you are successful.
- If you don't have any major health problems, you're successful.
- If you have a disease and you're in a wheelchair, however, you do not have a successful life.

My version of success is as follows:

- With love, disease is a powerful teacher that can show us all that we can push beyond our physical limitations and experience joy and abundance from a different place. It can come from somewhere inside of us, by knowing that we're whole and loving ourselves no matter what we look like or feel like or the circumstances of our life.

NO MAP REQUIRED

If you truly trust your life, then it doesn't matter where you're going or where you've been. You just have to start where you are. There's no prerequisite. No matter what is happening in your life, you're never off your path. Disease does not take you farther away from home. Lupus does not make you lost. Instead, it reminds you that you are whole. You are on track. You are where you are supposed to be.

CHOOSE IT

The most important aspect of trusting your life is simply choosing to do so. You have to *choose* to trust your life. You have to choose to believe that your life is going to work *for* you and not *against* you. You have to make that thought real in your mind. And if you struggle with that, then you need to at least invest in the concept that you want to trust your life. Until you actually believe it, you need to wake up every day and say, "My life is going to work for me and not against me."

If you have a disease, that means you choose to trust all of your life, including the disease. You have to choose the illness and the heartbreak and the beauty and the joy. You have to choose to trust homelessness or the nice house. You have to choose to trust your entire life. Choosing means trusting. Trusting means you're never off your path; everything that's coming into your life is here to help you grow, and you can't discount anything—you are 100 percent responsible for what shows up.

Choosing trust, choosing love—that action feeds us. A loving action will at first help our minds, but eventually, enough love and trust have the potential to help heal our physical bodies as well.

FORGET THE MOUNTAINTOP MOMENT

I have an opinion about climbing to the top of a mountain, then sitting and meditating until you're enlightened. I think it's a load of crap. I think we find enlightenment by living on the frontlines of life and by choosing a different way of thinking and framing every single time, all day long. It's like becoming a student to life.

Each time you have a struggle come toward you, instead of putting up the sword I want you to put your arms out and embrace it. Each time difficulty hits me, I ask the same question now: "What is the wisdom and loving coming forward with this event?" Then it has meaning. Then it has a place. Then the hard experiences bring wisdom. And yes, at first I am in shock when horribly painful things occur. And I allow myself to feel sad. But as I move through the experience now, I have a higher vantage point to look from, which is, "I trust that there may be some beautiful things about myself and my loving in this hard time I am having."

Embracing the struggle can make us more alive. It can be enlightening. And it can bring knowledge to us, because it shows us how to be more compassionate to ourselves instead of holding up a sword. You don't need to be meditating on a mountaintop to dig deep and gain knowledge. The best opportunities for knowledge arise from handling and embracing the most difficult circumstances we face.

Take, for example, a cancer diagnosis. Challenging, painful, and difficult? Yes. That's not a debate. But stop for a moment and consider turning that diagnosis into the richest, most full experience that you have had in your life. If you decide to believe it, then cancer can teach you something. It can teach you how to love yourself. It can teach you that you're still okay, even though something is impacting your body and doesn't feel good. It can teach you how to be good to others. It can show you how to get the life that you really want.

Another example is someone who has a heart attack and nearly dies. Maybe he quits his job and chases his dream of building the start-up company he's forever considered doing. Disease can be a pivotal moment in our life if we shift our perspective in the way we think about it. And chronic disease is a powerful teacher in that way. Because if we listen to what it's trying to teach us—and for everyone it's different—it can change our focus of how we want to live our life.

MY TURNING POINT

Before my life took a negative turn, I meditated every day. I practiced yoga and I went through the motions of what I thought it meant to be mindful. I thought I was a spiritual person. Then the sky started falling, and I got pushed down under water and I thought I was going to drown. That's when I decided to truly take a different approach. My situation was life circumstances, but illness has the same impact.

People don't change their life unless they get pushed off a cliff, right? Hard times cause us to consider different paths. I would not have discovered love as a healing tool unless I was suffering so horribly. So we humans can change things now, or we can wait to fall off the cliff. If you are reading this book, however, I bet you feel like you have gotten pushed off the cliff in some way in your life.

A LOVING AFFIRMATION

Everything is coming present for my upliftment. I am open to discovering the opportunities my life is presenting me.

10

FIND YOUR HELD BELIEFS
AND RELEASE THEM

We get to the loving
by taking a risk for ourselves.

♥

*M*y client Martha had dealt for years with a horrible bacterial infection called C. diff. She also had Hashimoto's. She battled C. diff for several years, having contracted it as a secondary infection at the hospital when she had her appendix removed. C. diff is hard to treat and can be antibiotic resistant. Martha was so knocked over by her C. diff infection, she couldn't take care of herself after she contracted it. And to make matters worse, she had a newborn baby at home. C. diff is a serious illness. It's immune suppressive. Martha had no energy, she couldn't walk, and she had bloody stool for endless months. She couldn't digest food and was in severe and serious pain. It literally wiped her out.

After simply existing with this illness for years—four or five— after doctors essentially told her there was nothing more they could do for her, Martha came to me. She and I worked together to change her outlook. She'd been following the AIP diet when she could eat, and she had done all that her doctors had instructed. The first thing I told her was what an amazing job she'd been doing living with this disease so far. Her circumstances were exceptional and she'd survived them. She'd also done something that was challenging for her: She had accepted help and love from people—mostly out of necessity, as she was unable to care *for herself. We talked through a lot of her challenges and what emerged was a clear understanding that she'd never thought herself worthy or deserving of people helping her, regardless of how difficult it was for her to function. Before C. diff Martha was a doer and a go-getter. She managed a lot of things. When this happened, she couldn't manage anything. She became almost helpless in the midst of having a newborn. She didn't really know how to believe it at first.*

We eventually talked about that worth and really worked on her understanding that she was worthy of accepting help and the generosity and kindness of others. C. diff helped Martha come to the conclusion she was worthy of people's help and love. What a wisdom giver! I assured her at this point that she didn't need to change anything. That love was hers to accept if she could just believe herself worthwhile. We also tried to examine the benefits and positives that arrived along with C. diff. Had it in any way made her life better? The answer was yes. Because of C. diff, Martha changed in the following ways:

- *She gathered and learned new skills.*
- *Her mothering skills became different.*
- *She learned that she was worthy of help.*
- *She stopped spending so much effort being an overachiever.*
- *She learned to work within the capacity of what her life gave her.*
- *Mostly, she grew happy with all that was thrown her way.*
- *She learned to trust that she was doing things "right," not failing the life test.*

Martha has removed the pressure of feeling she had to be a superwoman. It's changed her whole view of why she even got C. diff, because now she has more patience with herself, recognizing that she's doing the best that she can, and she really,

really understands this on a deep level now. That's a powerful weapon for her. She trusts her husband more. She trusts herself more. She trusts her friends more. She's taking her life one day at a time. What has emerged from all of this is believing in herself and believing that she's moving through her illness in the right way, or in a way that works for her. In the process, she came to find a medical option she might not have had the openness to discover.

There's a fairly new and slightly radical treatment for C. diff called fecal transplant, during which a patient is injected with stool from someone else. It's somewhat crude, new science, but big universities are starting to try it with great success. It floods the large intestine with large amounts of the beneficial bacteria found in healthy people. One drawback, in addition to being somewhat scary, is that it's expensive.

But once Martha made the decision that getting the bacterial infection actually had the potential to make her life better, the idea and opportunity of getting a fecal transplant manifested in her life. She quickly reached out to her doctor, and it was a very short process before she underwent the amazingly radical new treatment that has a high success rate. Once Martha felt aligned inside of herself and accepted C. diff, she started enjoying her life more in the midst of having this disease. That was when the disease itself shifted, and this whole new radical treatment came forward as an option in her life, which it never had before. She said that it had never been an option financially. Suddenly it was. She had always been too afraid to try something so radical, because she always feared that something would make her even sicker. With more trust in how she's working her health-care routine, she was able to do it. The end result: She trusted more fully that when an option came to her, she should examine it more carefully instead of being so scared about it.

CONSCIOUS BELIEFS VERSUS UNCONSCIOUS ONES

When something happens to us in our life, and we actually have an internal conversation in our minds about it, those are conscious thoughts or beliefs. For example:

- *Life is against me.*
- *Life is hard.*
- *I must have done something bad for this to happen to me.*
- *I don't deserve health.*

We all have conscious thoughts when something really hard is happening, because we need to make sense of it. Beliefs are made up because we have decided something about the world, usually through an experience that we've had in our life. For example, your father abandoned you. Your mother decided not to mother you. You were abused. You were beaten. You were bullied. It doesn't matter—it can be any negative or traumatic experience. They're all unique to our experience. We have a conscious thought right when those things happen to make sense of our world, such as, "Oh, my father is beating me. So I must not be worthy of love." We make up beliefs to survive in a harsh world, so that we can move on.

When we keep ourselves in alignment with those conscious thoughts, they become ingrained beliefs. They start as conscious thoughts that we have an investment in, because our investment is survival, and they move into the unconscious space because nothing happens with them. Eventually, because we haven't done anything to change them and we still believe them, they move into the unconsciousness and remain in our life. What started out as conscious moves into the unconscious, and then that moves from the unconscious into the body. That's where I see the root of illness. These principles of holding held beliefs are based on the work of Dr. Robert D. Waterman, EdD, LPCC, who created the modern-day Noetic Field Therapy practice. Noetic Field Therapy™ has its roots in the healing modalities created by Phineas Parkhurst Quimby and later expanded by Dr. Neva Dell Hunter.

UNCONSCIOUS BELIEFS GET IN THE WAY

Unconscious beliefs ultimately block our divineness. They block joy. Thankfully, since they are blocks to joy, they will eventually come forward as opportunities to finding that joy. Since we have to choose joy, the wisdom will come forward. Eventually realizations emerge. Thoughts like:

- *I really am deserving of loving.*
- *I really am deserving of health.*

If you hadn't had a problem come forward, then you wouldn't have been able to make the connections about what you deserve in life. You now have an opportunity here to enrich your life through the process of reflection.

Working with a Loving Diet practitioner can help you figure out your unconscious beliefs. That's the hard part of all this. Most people don't even know that their beliefs are holding them back. Some people don't even realize that they have a belief that they don't deserve love. Some people don't know that deep down they think that God has forgotten them or that they are not important enough. Those are common beliefs, too. Sometimes, just having the intention that you want to know what your unconscious beliefs are will help you get in touch with them. You can also work with a practitioner, who is skilled in this kind of energy work, and who can help you get in touch with your beliefs.

Let's return to the blob for a moment to try to access your beliefs on your own. When you talk to the blob, ask it what its gifts are. The gift can be the reverse of a held belief. You can review any moments in your life that were really difficult or traumatic and you can ask to be shown. If you aren't shown anything, invent something. Sometimes, even what we fabricate is true. There's no harm in forgiving a belief that doesn't exist within you. The important part is having the intention to uncover your held beliefs, and then, when you figure out what the beliefs are, you can say, "I forgive myself for believing that God had forgotten about me. I forgive myself for believing that I wasn't worthy of love."

Unconscious beliefs ultimately block our divineness. They block joy. Thankfully, since they are blocks to joy, they will eventually come forward as opportunities to finding that joy.

♥

CLEARING BELIEFS

There are three excellent ways for clearing beliefs that are blocking our divine nature and blocking health:

1. Forgiveness statement: Make a statement forgiving a belief you have.
2. Epiphanies: You can have epiphanies such as, "Oh, that isn't working," or you can, what I call, fake it till you make it.
3. Choosing: Choose to find what is holding you back. Choosing is an intention.

HOW TO: A FORGIVENESS STATEMENT

For a forgiveness statement, I'd like you to say to yourself or to me, "I forgive myself for believing that I'm not worthy." It's as simple as that. You simply complete a forgiveness statement. You can write it down, you can say it quietly to yourself, or you can say it in front of another person. When you repeat forgiveness statements, it is a rapid way of clearing held beliefs that you've made up about safety, security, and love in the world, based on circumstances in your life. When you bring a belief to the surface and place awareness upon it, then it can resolve rather quickly.

HOW TO: EPIPHANIES

Epiphanies just kind of happen. They're floating around, waiting for you to realize them. They can happen in yoga class when you suddenly hear that mantra you've been saying to yourself over and over and over again that's been so hopeful for you. Epiphanies often feel sudden. It's as if you can suddenly see something all the way through to the end that you couldn't see before. We all have epiphanies. Either they just land in our laps or we have a really emotional moment, like giving birth or falling in love—or we ask for them. You may have an epiphany when you realize that a prior event in your life made you feel unworthy of love.

During an epiphany, your unconscious, held beliefs may begin to come forward. As humans we're here to learn. We're here to have experiences that will help us uncover truths for ourselves and discover that the world is safe and that we are worthy of love. When we understand how what we believe about the world is not true, we get to change those beliefs. And that kind of experiential learning deepens our wisdom. So they are wonderful springboards for learning. We are all, by virtue of being born on the planet, worthy of love, worthy of health. We're worthy of safety and security.

So, in essence, when these issues come forward during an epiphany, we can work them out and be more connected to the loving inside of ourselves. We can then have abundant health, wealth, and happiness from the inner knowing that we're worthy of love, that the world is a safe place, and that the root of who we are is beautiful, loving, and divine. Our unconscious held beliefs only come forward in an epiphany to help us remember that.

HOW TO: CHOOSING

It's your choice. The crux of The Loving Diet is that your life can change, but you have to want to change it. You have to ask for it. It's an awakening process through intention, asking, and wanting. By virtue of picking up this book, you're probably open to it. Love is a non-inflicting energy. It will support anything you believe. So if you believe you are worthy, it shows up as worthy. If you believe you are a victim, it shows up as victim. The very root of this philosophy of loving is choice. You must ask love to come into your life. That is when it will. But it may not look like what you expect, so releasing judgments about what love looks like is important. Love can look like a job loss, so that the new job that is better can come forward. Love can look like a healing crisis. That is where the trust comes in. Ask for love, then trust what presents itself. Because you asked it from a loving place, what presents itself is for the highest good. And the highest good is the best-possible scenario.

Do you want your life to work for you? Or do you want your life to work against you? Say to yourself: *I want more love; I want more abundance; I want health; I want happiness; and I want my life to feel different than it feels right now.* That's the choosing.

A HELD BELIEF ABOUT LOVE

I'm friends with Tom, who was married for twenty years, and his wife was quite mean to him during a good part of their marriage. When he would come home at night, he felt like a punching bag for her unhappiness and anger about her own life. She would place lots of demands and high expectations on him to make her happy. He started making excuses for coming home late to avoid the conflict. He loved her, but he did not know how to make her happy. And in the process of trying to make her happy, his own happiness dwindled. Eventually, after exhausting every option, including therapy, he asked for a divorce. Now on his own in the world of being single, he's tapping into some big fears. He's afraid that because he loved once, and he thought she was the one, he won't be able to trust love again. After all, his wife wasn't mean to him when they first got together. But over time, her anger issues surfaced that were uncomfortable for everyone in the family, and he started to wonder how the woman he loved so much at first could be so different years later. How could he have chosen so poorly? And how could he trust not to make the same mistake again? Valid question!

He wondered post-marriage, "What am I going to do? Here I am, looking for love, and now I can't trust it. The vulnerability of love seems too intense. What if someone else looks to me for their happiness again?" There's one way to look at it, which is, "Wow. You really crashed and burned the first time you got married. You better hope it doesn't happen again," which seems like an easy and normal perspective to take. That worry left him feeling apprehensive about diving into the pool of love again, because who knew what was behind door number two? He almost didn't trust himself to say yes to letting love in again. He didn't trust himself to make a good decision—one that would protect him from making that mistake again. He didn't trust that he could tell the difference between real gold and pirate's gold when it came to love. And let me tell you, this guy is super smart and successful. He didn't have any problem figuring out solutions in other areas of his life. But this was a matter of the heart. His "failed" marriage made him scared to trust his ability to choose wisely again, or even if there was an amazing woman out there, would she be able to fully love him? That quandary created this question he carried around with him. This was due partly because he felt like his father never made him a loving priority growing up. His father was always preoccupied with himself. So he married a woman who did not make him a priority in her life and was a bit preoccupied with anger from her childhood. Can you see the perfect storm here? Another mistake seemed inevitable because he had chosen so poorly the first time, right?

The better perspective: He was tuned in enough to know that while he thought he'd found his soul mate, he could see it wasn't working. He had stopped trusting himself, stopped trusting that love would show up in a beautiful, caring way in the framework of his marriage. He wasn't caring for himself by staying in the relationship. But eventually he did care for himself by having the courage to call off the marriage and take steps to see if he could get that deep love he always longed for. He knew enough to know that rather than live a life of misery, he would need to get a divorce. Knowing that allowed him to lean into that wisdom and that insight. He had information on how relationships worked because he learned from one that did not work out. It's not confirmation that it won't happen again, but it's trust that he already had skills inside of him to know when it wasn't working—knowledge that might make a difference the next time around. The next big step in his life, after that kind of wisdom coming forward, is trusting his own vulnerability to move forward when the authentic love does appear at his doorstep. It is not that love will get easier; it actually may be scarier. But the wisdom doesn't leave us, and now he has the choice to decide if he will choose from a different perspective. If he does, then he gets the riches only authentic love can bring. And it comes from knowing he has it inside himself, and the loving he used to take care of his own heart. Big love on the inside of himself will draw big love on the outside.

His misguided belief: I'm not worthy of love and a long-lasting relationship.

The better perspective: I deserve amazing love because I didn't stay in a bad marriage.

EXERCISE:

Find Held Beliefs

Consider working with someone to help you understand and examine your held beliefs. In the meantime, set an intention. Write it down now in a notebook. Ask yourself what's holding you back. Think back to childhood, college, whatever and whenever, recalling situations. Free-form writing is a great way to draw out thoughts. Just write in a journal. Don't think about it or edit. Just write and see what comes up. Read a week's worth of journaling at the end of each week and see what comes up. Also, keep repeating that intention. It will emerge eventually, potentially in indirect ways.

A LOVING AFFIRMATION

I trust my life to show me what's working and not working for my highest good.

11

LOVE WHAT IS PRESENT

Illness is the wave.
Love is the ocean.

AUTOIMMUNE DISEASE ISN'T CURABLE. That means that in some form or another it will be present with you for your life. You get to choose if this fact is going to add to your life or take away from your life. My philosophy: The disease and the struggle are here anyway, so why not make the most of them?

I feel suffering, and I feel it on many days, but I still have a deep, deep trust that whatever is presenting itself is for my upliftment—that there's some kind of wisdom in it for me that's going to help my life. There are some tools that help, such as the food plan, which you'll soon learn to use, but finding the trust and the love comes with meditation. Forgiveness statements, ancient Hawaiian practices, and more are also in my kit and should be in yours, too.

PRACTICAL TOOLS TO EASE SUFFERING

Because I have known suffering, I want to pass along some tools I use when I am feeling hopeless. Most likely what you're dealing with—if you do have autoimmune disease—is not curable. You'll need to learn to trust it, embrace it, and work through it. I hope the tools in *The Loving*

Diet provide you with help and that you find a bit of use from them. And know that if I could hold your hand, I would.

1. Give yourself thirty minutes and go into the pain. Really, the center of our suffering is a bit like the eye of a hurricane. If you take a moment to go right into the most painful part, relief may come. Breathe it in. Breathe in that very, very hard piece you are trying to run away from. Pull it close to you, and relax your body if you can. Just keep breathing into it again and again. Let whatever comes up be there with you. Just focus on your breathing. See if you can manage this for fifteen- to twenty-minute increments.

2. Go to bed two hours earlier than usual. I go to bed around 8:30 or 9:00 p.m. when I am in pain. It helps to regulate cortisol. Plus, the body needs a tremendous amount of metabolic energy to manage pain of any kind. So while you are in the thick of it, sleep often. And here is the thing: Pain in the heart can cause pain in the body. Pain in the body can cause pain in the heart. It isn't important how or why you are suffering.

3. Try taking ignatia amara. Some call this the Homeopathic Prozac. Awesome. Hand it over. This remedy is wonderful for grief, anxiety, insomnia, headaches, and hopelessness. It is the most classic grief remedy in homeopathic medicine. Think sorrow. Think crying. Think sadness from some kind of big upheaval. Hallmarks also include sighing a lot, crying while alone, and feeling emotionally sensitive. You will need a homeopath to help you with the dose, but 200C twice per day may be a good starting point.

4. Let yourself be sad. Give yourself permission to feel grief. Say it out loud: "I give myself permission to be sad" or "I am doing a great job letting myself be sad today." This is a very important piece of suffering. When you are upset about your circumstances, it can make those around you feel uncomfortable. Don't let that

deter you. The more you walk toward what ails you, the more quickly you will come out the other side.

5. Keep a journal. Write down what you are feeling every day. Writing can be an effective tool for dealing with traumatic events. Or write a letter to your disease telling it how you really feel about it. Let it rip. Then burn the letter.

6. Change the scenery. It will help keep you from stagnating. Even if it is a short trip to your favorite store. Don't overdo it; too much could make you more tired. But little breaths of fresh air help.

7. Be more thoughtful about how you manage your diet. Don't forget to eat. It's easy to forget when you're in the midst of sadness, grief, or suffering. Or the opposite. If you turn to food to help ease your suffering, call it out. Say to yourself, "I don't need food to help ease my suffering. I can do this." A balanced food intake will help manage cortisol.

8. Be sure you are digesting your meals. Stress contributes to low hydrochloric acid production in the stomach. So consider talking to your health-care practitioner to find a supplement that may assist with digestion if you need one.

9. Trust your life. There is something pushing your life forward that you may not be aware of yet. And if you don't trust it, and you hate everything, be okay with that, too. Being human is very, very, very hard some days. I jokingly text my girlfriends: *It was an especially hard day to be human today.* We have a good laugh. But you can trust life. This I know.

10. Trust your tenderness. It will get you more in your life than less. This is a hard one for me personally. I become tenderer by the

day doing this kind of work. And loving your life and your struggles may make you tenderer as well. I sometimes think I speak a language only a few understand in the physical realm. It can be a hard buy-in to choose the tender route. Do it anyway and do not hesitate. I would rather get broken a thousand times than stay safe in my protective cocoon and not experience the richness of life.

If I have to go out in the world teary-eyed from it all, then I will. Being vulnerable to life is the ticket to great love of ourselves and our life. It may level the playing field, but know the players you surround yourself with are the bravest of the bunch. The ones who choose to go big. Those are the ones I want to invest in.

We can say our suffering is so potent because we are attached. But it is natural to suffer when we receive a diagnosis or news of some sort we don't want to. It is deep work to accept our disease. It is profound work to become friendly and loving toward what ails us. I do believe it can be done. I do believe there is a vast resource at our fingertips in the midst of suffering.

TOOLS FOR LOVING WHAT IS PRESENT

There are many ways to learn to love what is present—tools you can rely on every day. At first, these tools might not come easily to you, but choose small things such as being nice to the grocery store cashier or appreciating someone in your family even if they aren't supportive. Wrap your mind around the small stuff before you try tackling the big stuff.

1) LOVE THE SADNESS

This is challenging, because we have to trust that we won't get lost in our sadness. We have to trust that some wisdom will come forward to serve us in some way when we become sad. We have to trust that we're going to make it out the other side. The only way to unravel sadness is to go into it.

For a lot of people it's enough to feel sad and then that will unwind itself. For some people, getting through the sadness is more difficult. Some need a counselor for the larger issues they're working through. Some need to create structure around it. Others need to accept that sadness wave when it rolls in and be quiet for a moment with their sadness—maybe blink an extra time, practice an extra meditation, or go to yoga class.

Here are a few ways you can better love and accept your sadness:

- Create a space base—a time and place to be sad. Define when you'll be sad if you can't be sad all the time.
- Surround yourself with loving people who will assist you as you move through the sadness.
- Recognize that sadness is a normal part of being human.
- Believe that it is okay to trust sadness.
- Acknowledge that the more you let sadness be with you, the quicker you will get out of it.

When we open our hearts to the natural process of sadness, we move through it the quickest way possible. We learn that we can gain wisdom that will help our lives, and that the process is going to benefit us in some way. We're well equipped to do this. Look at children and how they react when they're upset about something. They don't push away sadness until they're taught to later in life. Take, for example, a couple of five-year-old children playing. One of them grabs the toy out of the other's hand. The other one starts crying because he's sad about it. As teens, it's a different story: When someone steals a boyfriend, the behavior turns more passive-aggressive. As an adult, sometimes we react to a cancer diagnosis with anger, meanness, or blame, instead of just being sad.

2) MEDITATION

Meditation is a form of relaxation, focus, and centeredness. It's about creating stillness both in your body and mind. Some people find it challenging to stop the stirring in their heads. But once you can find a way to do it, the benefits are enormous. Once you figure it out, it becomes easier to be present.

I meditate anywhere I can find time. Usually, I carve out twenty-five minutes from my day. I don't do anything fancy. I sit down, set my timer, and watch my breath. My mind of course talks to me, but I keep refocusing on my breath. If you find a place in your area that offers meditation practice, I encourage you to sign up—especially as you get started. It is great to learn with a group. Many of my friends meditate with others in a group setting. You can search for meditation groups near you. In fact, many hospitals now offer meditation classes. Working within the context of a group will increase your confidence to establish a practice you can do on your own. I have meditated now for over a decade. I can sit anywhere if I have even a few minutes and calm myself by meditation. I even meditate while I am at the dentist (along with a progressive muscle relaxation exercise). You can meditate at home, in your car, or wherever you can sneak the time to sit.

LEARNING TO MEDITATE

- Join a class online or in your community.
- Check out great online meditation classes offered by Oprah and Deepak Chopra.
- Set aside twenty-five minutes per day.
- Consider attending a two- or three-day meditation retreat.
- Buy a book on meditation.
- Know that meditation does not inflict on religious beliefs. It is a form of relaxation.

Find a minimum of ten to twenty-five undisturbed minutes. Sit comfortably. Close your eyes and breathe slowly. Follow your breath—work on visualizing it going in and out. That's meditation and that's enough to change the hard wiring of your brain. You can try this in the bathtub, in a room you designate, or on the couch; just find the time away from any distractions and know that there is no right or wrong way to do it. The only wrong way is not doing it at all.

Ideally, I'd like you to find twenty-five minutes a day to meditate. That's the golden number. Once you feel comfortable and have mastered following your breath, then take it one step further. Silently, in your mind, ask for love. Ask the universe to bring more loving into your life. That's the way I meditate now—with a call to the universe that says I want my life to have more loving in it. I'll be honest, too: I'm busy. I often try to cheat the system. That means I do my twenty-five minutes in the car between errands. And that's okay—as long as you do it.

As you get deeper into your meditation practice, you can add a visualization element. I see the love coming in from the high heavens and the earth, and each time I take in a breath, I picture it then entering the top of my head and my feet. With every breath I take, I fill my heart with love. I fill my body with loving inside from the outside. That visualization creates a strong physical sensation. But be detached from the form in which the loving arrives. It may not show up in the expected form. Don't worry: Regardless of how it shows up, you're still on track.

*M*y client Jody has irritable bowel syndrome (IBS). She works a stressful job at a finance company. She is also a mom of two kids under ten. She began meditating after we worked together, and she started on a low-inflammatory diet. She knew her stress was a big culprit in her IBS flares. Each morning she would wake up fifteen minutes before her prior wake-up time to mediate. At first it was difficult to keep her attention on her breath. But after a few weeks, she noticed an immediate calming *effect. In fact, if she was in traffic, instead of feeling the gripping stress of getting home late, she would practice following her breath instead. And when her boss would walk into her office and start making demands on her, she would silently watch her breath to stay calm. She noticed her flare decreased as a result of managing her stress and diet differently. She was able to work with her doctor to lower her medications as a result of her new-found healing resource.*

Something Big Will Emerge

Let's do this together (and do it again later when you can close your eyes).

- Take a deep breath. Now in your mind, picture what your illness looks like and feels like. It probably has a very definitive, energetic feeling for you of hatred. You hate it, or you're frustrated by it, most likely.
- Use whatever you feel for your illness to visualize it. Do you have a picture of it in your mind? If you can, take a couple of deep breaths. Now one more. And then, as you exhale, think of something you love—your children, a retreat spot that makes you happy, whoever or whatever brings love to you. Think about that love for a moment. Think about how that feels—find a tender moment to envision it.
- Now, hold on to that feeling, and let's do a little experiment. Take that feeling and transfer it to the illness. Love it. Think of how your children are just the best thing ever; now apply that same tenderness to the illness. Trade the love for your family or your happy place with your illness and apply that loving feeling. That's it. I'm not asking you to do anything else or make any decisions, just to be tender toward what you are mostly used to disliking. Can you do that? Can you feel a sensation—and maybe even find a beautiful part to this illness?

- It's not easy. I'm asking you to love the entire part of you. Everything that's making you up right now. You're having a loving thought about it—feeling connected and loving inside of yourself—loving the illness like you love your family. Loving all of you.

- Take it one step further: What if this disease didn't hold you back? What if you knew you could move through it to something better on the other side of it? What does that other side look like to you? It's something different, I know that much. I'm asking you to ask your brain to do something that it is not used to doing, in part because maybe the illness represents weakness or failure to you. Disconnect from that for a moment. Don't let the mind spin. Say what you need to say, but move your attention down into your chest.

- Then take one more deep breath, moving that into your chest. You can even stop thinking about the illness, but think of who you are as a whole right now, in this moment, exactly all of the atoms and molecules that you consist of, the outfit that you're wearing, how your hair looks today . . . everything right now. There's a completeness that you already have. There's a deeper wisdom coming forward through this illness that has something to tell you.

A Broader Coping Mechanism

When you are really suffering or are jammed up in a particular situation, take many meditation moments, whenever you can, and ask to be shown the way. Take deep breaths and ask for more loving. You might do this for thirty seconds and you'll feel good for a minute, but then immediately you're back in the pit. That's okay; do it again. In my darker moments, I stop and do this mini-meditation forty times a day.

Your perspective will eventually change, even though the situation remains the same. You'll start to realize that nothing is off track, the timing is right, and your life is right. You might not have the tools to immediately fix your illness, but you'll be able to alter your perspective on how you deal with it, and from there, all sorts of wonderful things occur.

Remember:

- This is how it's supposed to be right now.
- Everything is okay.
- You can trust the timing of your life.
- You can trust what is happening right here and right now.
- You're not off of anything.
- You don't need to get anywhere, go anywhere.
- Everything is okay right now, the way it is.
- You are okay.

Your perspective will eventually change, even though the situation remains the same. You'll start to realize that nothing is off track, the timing is right, and your life is right.

♥

Whatever you're dealing with, it is exactly the way it's supposed to be, and I'm so sorry that it feels like you're struggling—but you're actually not. If you just accept this right now, this not knowing where you're supposed to be, then the suffering automatically eases up. If you can't get your head around this yet in terms of the illness being what it is supposed to be, replace "illness" with something else that's frustrating you or causing you pain in life. Fixing the perspective is applicable in any situation. When I first started on The Loving Diet, I inched along. I failed at it all the time. I thought, *Oh, I got relief for twenty seconds*, and then my mind would start telling me things again, such as, *You're not worthy of love because your husband cheated on you and left you. You're just a piece of crap.* Your mind might instead say things like, *Oh, this disease is going to kill you,* or, *Something is not right because you have Hashimoto's.*

Think about those twenty seconds. Over a period of time, they keep building. After a while, even if you're not free from that suffering caused by your illness, your life is whole and you have a framework within which to work. Those twenty seconds, over and over, will have built confidence and trust in you. Eventually, even though you are suffering, you'll develop trust in your life.

3) YOU DON'T NEED TO GO OUTSIDE YOURSELF

Love is instantaneous, but you have to ask for it. That's another cool aspect about it. Love isn't related to most of the things we think we need. *I need to go to spin class. I need to count calories. I need to buy different clothes.* Those are things that are outside of yourself to solve. Ask for the love first.

4) UNCOVERING INNER WISDOM

You are amazing. You are truly amazing. The illness may try to knock you off your center, but repeat to yourself, "No, I have all the answers inside of me. I am an amazing person." The illness is testing you so that you will lean into something deeper that will help you in a different way in your life. You already have this place inside of you that you go to, and the world might try to tell you differently, but the illness is trying to help you remember something about yourself. It's not about the illness; it's about something else.

5) HO'OPONOPONO

In addition to meditation, I used Ho'oponopono, an ancient Hawaiian technique of resolution and forgiveness, which in turn acts as an energetic clearer. It was used by Hawaiians to resolve situations. The premise of Ho'oponopono is taking responsibility by saying, "I love you. I'm so sorry we had to do it this way. Please forgive me. I love myself." You can practice it with someone present or without.

When I'm in conflict with an issue or a person, I close my eyes and I think, *I'm so sorry we had to do it this way. Please forgive me. I love you and I love myself.* It helps to resolve conflict because it resolves it inside of yourself. Forgiveness provides that release.

This technique is a great way to clear held beliefs or to work on our relationships with other people, like our husbands, our wives, our loved ones, our mothers, our fathers. Often, these beliefs are integrated somehow in our disease and our beliefs about and toward our disease. Most times working with clients, there is a held belief connected with their physical illness. It can be a traumatic event like a parent dying, or abandonment, or something simple like a friend leaving their life. Whatever the case, to make sense out of the hurt or upset, we decide something about our life. What we decide about life isn't true; it is only a belief we made up to make sense of the hard thing we experienced. So if your father abandoned the family growing up, you may have decided as a child that people you love are not dependable. Or if your mother passed away from cancer when you were in college, you may have decided that loving people isn't safe because they could leave you. There may come a time when you happen upon these beliefs. Usually this occurs in a time of suffering, because of your willingness to get to the bottom of something that isn't serving you so that you can have more happiness in your life. That is where The Loving Diet comes in. Because just as important as changing your diet are your beliefs about life. They can be as limiting as eating gluten when you have celiac. So when you start discovering beliefs that you hold that no longer serve you, or block the joy of your loving heart, you can use forgiveness statements to clear them. You can say:

- "I forgive myself for believing loving someone isn't safe."
- "I forgive myself for believing God forgot about me when I got my MS diagnosis."

- "I forgive myself for believing that I am not worthy of good health or healing."

After you say a forgiveness statement, you can take a deep breath and let go. Often when clients repeat forgiveness statements and clear a big chunk of blocked energy, they feel lighter, brighter, and more hopeful. This is similar to a standard forgiveness statement, but this may resonate more with you. I personally use both forgiveness statements and Ho'oponopono. This method works well when others are involved, as opposed to a forgiveness statement, which is more about your unconscious beliefs.

I use Ho'oponopono as part of The Loving Diet because almost everyone has someone in his or her life with whom he or she still has issues. If you feel like you still have issues, practice Ho'oponopono, because then it's simply one more item you can check off the list that might be holding back good health for you.

6) THE BENEFIT OF REFRAMING YOUR LIFE

Why is reframing important? Reframing is important because it can be the most powerful evidence that life is working for you, not against you. Take, for example, Nelson Mandela, who spent all those years in prison. He used that time to write, pray, forgive, and come to peace. So would you say his prison sentence was useless? Well, you could theorize that he could have done all those things if he wasn't in prison, too. But we don't know that for sure. What we do know is that some of his most important work as a human—examining his life and growing his heart—was done in captivity. So judging the captivity (or in your case the illness) isn't going to get you closer to the cure. What will is cooperating with your circumstances and opening your heart to whatever is going to present itself. Nelson Mandela had no idea he would become President of South Africa. But what he did know in jail was that his own mind was the biggest prison of all. You have the same choice he did. Lift and love using what is present in your life as a tool of transformation. But you have to choose to.

Consider reframing your situation and thinking:

- *I'm going to use my disease to get the life I want.*
- *I'm going to use multiple sclerosis to springboard into enjoying my life and trusting it and knowing that I'm okay even though I have MS.*
- *Cancer is helping me become a more loving person.*

REFRAME IT

When you see yourself going down the rabbit hole of "why me," "oh no," or "I hate this," don't judge yourself. That is a normal, human response. Use those phrases as reminders that you don't feel comfortable with life right now and see what happens when you surrender to those feelings and visualize what might be on the other side of those feelings of frustration. For example, if you have tried and tried to get a job, and every time you don't you say, "I was rejected. They didn't pick me," let that be your reminder to continue on with that thought, "... but I also know I am doing a great job trying, I am learning to be humble and to trust life, and something will eventually come forward for me." You don't try to push away the *I was rejected* thought; you use it as a trigger to say something in addition to that statement, something that will work for you. See? Stumbling block to stepping stone. Use everything in life. You are doing this right. It is like a new muscle you are learning to flex.

My Reframing Experience

For me, struggle is struggle. It doesn't matter if you are dealing with an autoimmune disease, broken heart, cancer diagnosis, betrayal, or grief. All of those scenarios can cause a person to ask herself the same questions or make observations that may include: *Why is this happening; how can I stop feeling this way; why is there suffering in the world; why does life seem so unfair?*

When my husband and I split three years ago, we lived in our super-modern dream house on fifty acres. Surrounded by a fantastic community and loads of friends, I truly thought we would be together forever. Then "disaster" struck. He abruptly left, moved in with another woman he had been with for some unknown amount of time, and suddenly we could not keep the house while separated due to the high mortgage payment. I was suddenly incapacitated from heartbreak, was losing my dream home, was scrambling to understand what was happening, had a bewildered and sad six-year-old I was taking care of most of the time, and had not a clue about how to deal with any of it. This was not the plan I had signed up for. Or so I believed then. I thought my life had crumbled in an instant. Overnight, I started comparing myself to others. I looked at happy families, happy marriages in beautiful homes, and deemed them successful at life and myself unsuccessful. I know the same happens with illness. I listen to my clients' stories of ill health (mostly autoimmune disease), and there are a lot of conclusions that the world is a hostile place. What I did not know then was that this was the magic ticket to loving myself, having compassion for my struggles, and learning the power of forgiveness.

How many of you have had a heartbreaking or traumatic event? You get a diagnosis, accident, divorce, death, or loss of some kind. Life changes. A lot of "why is this happening to me" surfaces. So I allowed myself to ask that question. A lot. I let myself feel sad for a long time. I dedicated days and months to crying. And in those days and months of sadness, I suffered from waves of regret, bitterness, fear, humility, and finally peace. Out of this ordeal came the conclusion that life is never broken, life is never off track, blessings are cleverly disguised as trage-dies, and every human being is privy to the riches of life.

In this process I was able to learn some valuable lessons that I have incorporated into my daily life as best I can. They were pivotal moments that changed my life, molecules, energy, and beliefs in an instant and provided fertile ground to use my "disaster" to be my blessing of untold measure. It had nothing to do with my diet, my supplements, my surroundings, or my lifestyle. It had to do with how I framed my situation. It became a change in my personal mantra for life. It is a practice, however, and like all humans, I am prone to the occasional pitfalls of negative self-talk. Through my experience, I awoke to the possibility that the universe was conspiring toward my wholeness. I began to let go more often of judging my disaster as bad and began to re-label it as my own personal blessing the universe created for my upliftment. It is hard to say the diagnosis of a disease or life as you know it falling apart could be a blessing, but perhaps this reframing of your thoughts could be a valuable exercise to consider.

Three Ways to Reframe Difficulty

1. How you approach your difficulty is the medicine. Ask yourself how you feel about your difficulty. You may think, *I am going to fight this disease. I am going to make that person pay for the pain they caused me. I am going to survive this. I am a survivor. I am a victim.* Everyone has a personal answer.

Now try an exercise to reframe your attitude toward your circumstances. I like to sit quietly and do this. Take a few breaths to relax and then pretend there is no good or bad about your situation. Pretend that there is a gift-giving universe behind your difficulty. Pretend for a moment that there is something about your difficulty that is a tailor-made blessing that at its very core is upliftment. See if you get a sense of what yours may be. It may look like this:

- Old thought: *I am so unlucky that I have multiple sclerosis. Life sucks. I am in pain often and feel like life is unfair.*
- New thought: *I am able to meet all my challenges as they come with humor and grace. I feel thankful for discovering how strong*

my heart is through this experience. I'm thankful for how much more gentle I am with myself now.

Or this:

- Old thought: *I am so pissed I can't eat the way I used to. It is so hard to spend money on all this food for this stupid new diet. I hate being sick.*
- New thought: *I am incredibly lucky this healing diet came forward in my life. I am a more loving and compassionate person now that I have to focus more on myself and my health. I am amazed at how quickly my body is healing with this new approach to wellness.*

I have completed these exercises and taped them on my mirror in the bathroom. I am a believer in "fake it till you make it." And when I imagine myself whole, being pulled forward in life by grace and abundance, I feel better. My constant reframing of my belief that it is grace and abundance pulling me forward, and not suffering and heartbreak, means that the universe is meeting me with just that. This takes practice. I am vigilant about this practice, as I consider it to be the important aspect of my health.

2. Appreciate what is present. Recently, I was feeling competitive toward someone. I felt the old pull of *Why can't I just be accepted?* So when I feel that lack of being accepted, I find that the universe keeps creating scenarios of being accepted over and over again, until I start reframing my belief to include *I am enough already*, and I can love and bless the person I feel competitive toward. *I change my relationship to the difficulty and let it become my medicine.* Health and healing are truly a multi-layered approach. All the things that manifest in my life get equal billing. Rejection, pain, suffering, euphoria, joy, healing . . . all of it

is coming forward so that I can be loving toward it. I have stopped pushing difficulty away as I see its potential to change how loving I can be in a matter of an instant. When I had to meet with lawyers about my divorce, I was so sad. I went to work sad and crying. For a moment, I felt weak. Then I reframed it. My clients may have appreciated how open-hearted I was that day. How compassionate I am to myself when I struggle. How thankful I am to have a friendship now with my ex. I spent the day appreciating how tender I was. I appreciated the lawyer having a box of tissues in his office. I appreciated how well my ex and I got along. I appreciated the Crock-Pot dinner I had made in anticipation of being sad and not wanting to cook after meeting with the lawyer.

3. Be gentle and loving to yourself. This may be the most difficult of them all. How many of you find it easier to be loving and gentle to others more than yourself? When I am gentle and loving to myself, then I am more able to be gentle and loving to others. Here is an example. You go to the grocery store and forget something important on your list. You return home and realize you forgot it.

- Old thought: *I am so mad at myself. That was so stupid of me. I'm really upset. I needed that ingredient to make dinner. Now everyone will be disappointed. I hate that my brain doesn't work well with my illness.*
- New thought: *Well, good thing I have frozen soup in the freezer to heat up tonight! Look how well that worked out! It must not have been the night for baked chicken. I feel upset at myself, but everyone messes up. This is a good reminder to start leaving that pad of paper in my purse so I can remember my grocery list, instead of depending on my brain, which occasionally takes a break from its duties.*

My good friends and family know that my biggest "disaster" has really been the most beautiful experience I have had. The very experience I thought would destroy me has allowed me to be a more loving person toward myself and my circumstances. It has taught me to reframe my circumstances and my struggles and transform my life into an adventure of my heart.

A LOVING AFFIRMATION

I believe in myself. I believe everything happening in my life is bringing me closer to wholeness, not further away.

12

YOUR LIFE IS YOUR OWN— LET ILLNESS CREATE OPPORTUNITY

The disease is the cure.

♥

EVERYONE HAS HIS OR her own process to endure; there are varying degrees of how much life pushes us into a corner of what we can do with it and what we can't or what's fair or not fair. You own your life—100 percent of it. That means taking responsibility for it.

We should always start with ourselves—loving ourselves, investing in loving our path. In doing so, you're creating a larger container for yourself, and every day you're filling up your own container. And when a container gets so filled that it starts spilling out and over, we meet others in the overflow. That is a wonderful connection because then we're not meeting people on the scarcity front. Don't spend all of your time and energy asking:

- What's wrong with me?
- What don't I have?
- What does everyone else have that I don't?
- What am I lacking?

Those are all places where we go outside of ourselves. Instead, love within yourself and your wholeness, and then there's no other place you need to be. Then the overflow brings opportunity and new ideas and people.

HOLLY'S HAPPINESS APPROACH

A woman named Holly contacted me. She had been diag-nosed with ulcerative colitis when she was twenty years old, following a colonoscopy. She had just graduated from high school. At the time, she was young and didn't know what to do with her life. In addition to just getting ready to embark on being an adult, she had this disease to contend with. For all sorts of reasons, she felt scared. The illness meant that she had bloody stool and generally felt crappy. She had lived with this for years. All that time, she suffered through her illness, doing exactly what doctors told her. She asked often if diet would stop the blood in her stool but was told it wouldn't. Frustrated, she did her own research and came up with a list of supple-ments. By the time she got around to calling me many years later, she had gotten married and had three kids whom she home-schooled. In addition to wanting to know what she could take and eat, she really wanted to know how to stop being so angry about the disease. She's the perfect example of someone in need of The Loving Diet—all factors coming into play to in-crease her wisdom and happiness. Eventually, she became open to tackling it all. We took the three-pronged approach of The Loving Diet.

1) MEDICAL

We reviewed the supplements she'd researched. I adjusted her list, told her what to take instead, and reviewed her doctor's notes and tests. Remember: We are working in conjunction with medical professionals through all of this. My goal with supplements was to heal her gut. She started taking special probiotics for the bacterial overgrowth in her small intestine. The goal was to get the bloody area to stop bleeding. We drew up the physiological piece of the puzzle and got her a plan.

2) DIET

I put Holly on the food portion of The Loving Diet for six weeks after she'd spent the previous six months on AIP without success. She took supplements to heal her gut and change the bacterial flora in her upper small intestine.

3) LOVE

Emotionally, Holly felt:

- Overwhelmed
- Angry
- Sad

As soon as we started to talk about all that she'd been through, Holly began to cry. She'd carried the emotional burden of the disease for years and years. She felt embarrassed that she cried. I told her to cry through it, that it was okay to get that out of the way and move through the sadness—that it's quickest if you let the tears come out.

We reframed her viewpoint of the disease, too:

- Ulcerative colitis is going to benefit your life.
- You are a mother of three kids; your three kids are going to come to you with some pretty big things that are going to be happening in their life.
- You have the ability now because you've gone through this, and you know what it's like to struggle, to have so much more compassion than you ever thought you could, and now you will understand when your kids are struggling, too. You'll be able to meet them on a completely different level than you ever could have if you hadn't had the ulcerative colitis.

We talked about ways that she could cry about a time in her life to feel the sadness. And that the sadness was really holding back the healing, because sadness takes up residence inside our body, inside our psyche, and inside our mind.

Holly learned to:

- Trust the sadness to come forward; it's not going to drown her.
- Have faith that it's not going take over her life.
- Believe that life isn't going to fall apart.
- Allow this space to come forward and feel the sadness.

That's a loving action: allowing ourselves to be sad. It's better to get up every day and say, "I'm sad today and look at how well I'm being sad," instead of getting up every day and saying, "I'm not supposed to be sad. I can't get a lot of work done when I'm sad." All I ask of anyone is to consider taking time out of each day to appreciate how hard you are working, and if letting the sadness in is too scary, then don't. But at least consider the idea of what it would be like if you did.

EXERCISE

Spend a Moment or Two Each Day with Your Sadness

When you're driving to the grocery store and the kids are in the backseat of the car, and you have two minutes to yourself as you drive, say to yourself:

- I'm going to be okay if I'm sad.
- I'm sad right now, and this illness is sad.
- I don't have all the answers today, but I'm trying.
- That's okay.
- I forgive myself.
- I forgive myself for believing that sadness is going to destroy my life.

❤   ❤   ❤

Hopefully by now you are considering a different resource for healing: love. You understand the importance of medicine and your doctor in your process. Now, as you learn to eat in order to heal, remember to come at it from a place of love, not lack. And remember that all three prongs of The Loving Diet—the medical, the love, and the food—are all tools at your disposal and all work together with you at the helm.

A LOVING AFFIRMATION

I am the author of my life. I trust myself to make loving decisions about my health care.

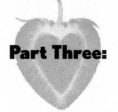

Part Three:

FOOD

Real nourishment equals

loving yourself.

13

THE LOVING DIET FOOD PROTOCOL

You were born, so you get
rock star status.

♥

AS WE ENTER THE food phase of The Loving Diet, I want to emphasize how important it is to approach this as not only a shift in the food you eat but also as *one part* of all three prongs of this program—medical, love, and food. It's difficult to start from where you are and change how you eat, regardless of how you approach it. But consider this: Since I specialize in this area, what I have found to be true—and this is one of the reasons why I developed The Loving Diet—is that at least half (if not more) of my clients are 100 percent compliant to the Autoimmune Paleo Diet and still not feeling as good as they hoped. I could walk into their AIP kitchen and see that there is nothing they're doing wrong; yet, they're not improving as much as they thought they would. That was what initially encouraged me to start thinking that there's more going on, that there's something else to people's feelings. If my clients are using medicine, looking at physiology, tracking their inflammation markers, changing their diet, taking the right supplements, and they're still not feeling better, there's another piece at play here, which is the relationship to their life. Sometimes, that relationship creates the belief that illness is here to destroy them. Or in a hidden place inside of themselves, they don't feel deserving of health or healing. Or they are not stepping forward out of being a victim of their illness, and their disease is still defining them rather than defining themselves by the amount of love in their life. Those are the people who find me: the ones who are not getting better on the AIP diet and are looking for a deeper context to define their health journey. That is the group I work for: the ones ready and willing to really get to work and go into the heart of their healing.

WHY PHYSICAL HEALTH IS ONLY PART OF THE PROGRAM

*O*ne of my clients, a woman named Sarah, gave me probably twenty pages of lab work (by the way, that much lab work is normal for my clients to give me!). She was 100 percent compliant on AIP, she took supplements, and I was probably the fourth or fifth practitioner she'd seen, including doctors. She had been to the best medical doctors and the best alternative doctors (including the top Paleo doctors) in the United States. At first I thought, What more could I possibly add to what she has already done? She had seen the best doctors! But we did work together, because Sarah discerned immediately that I take a different approach than most practitioners, and she was dedicated to improving her health.

Two or three sessions in, Sarah still wasn't feeling better, so I double-checked everyone's work; no one was missing anything. She had really severe blood sugar issues and we started talking about it. Because so much of my work with clients is intuitive, and energy work is a big part of The Loving Diet practice, when her father came up during one of our sessions, I asked, "Does your father have blood sugar issues?" She said, "That's so weird that you asked, because yes, he does." I said, "What was it like growing up with your dad?" Sarah told me that he was a hypercritical person who was miserable, and he told her she would amount to nothing, just like him. There it is.

He had a belief that she would amount to nothing and never tried hard enough (which really was his issue to work out; he just passed it along to her because that was the reality he lived in), and so not only did she buy into that belief but also she was mimicking her dad's physiology, because naturally she wanted his love, attention, and approval. For years, he'd told her that there was nothing she could do to be a winner in life and so her health became a reflection of that belief. Really that was a reflection of what he thought about himself, but it was passed on to Sarah, and ultimately there is wisdom in that false belief. She was now able to come to the conclusion that she was good enough and worthy of love, by having this karma with her father.

We started to reframe her destructive beliefs. Until that point, her dad had been a bit shut down and abrasive. She wondered if he loved her, and she was constantly fighting against the belief of being lovable, by creating relationship scenarios in her own life that would help her ultimately see that she was worthy of love. Built upon the relationship with her father, a shadow followed her around telling her that she was never going to amount to anything, that she was never going to deserve the riches of what love had to offer. The reframing looked like this: Sarah's dad was coming forward to help her work that out—that she was worthy of love. We went in and we started dissolving some held beliefs that she had around love and worthiness and people choosing her. That was done by choosing herself, her self-care, her own love for herself being the strongest medicine she could find. In that place, Sarah was able to find forgiveness for her father, acknowledge how difficult it had been for her growing up, and recognize that the constant relationship struggles with men and her health ultimately were there for her own benefit of wisdom.

End result: Sarah's health improved right away. Her blood sugar issues began resolving, her adrenal gland started regulating, and she began sleeping at night. She still went through some

*deeper emotional processes. This work tends to open up some-
one's life, so that he or she can start processing things and then
let them go. Sometimes it can look like things are getting a little
bit worse, but they're actually getting better. It just feels like
they're getting worse. Their relationships can get strained; there
might be an upset at work. But what's happening is that people's
lives are reworking themselves. It can be uncomfortable, but a
support team is good to have on hand to help with that. Some
people get immediate results, some people have miraculous healings—a miraculous healing being nothing more than an act of
love toward one's self.*

HOW TO FOLLOW THE LOVING DIET FOOD PROTOCOL

Depending upon your situation, the food protocol can be difficult, because you often have to give up some of your favorite foods. When you're
feeling frustrated, try to remember that you are doing this to try to improve your health. And isn't that worth giving up a slice of pizza or some
ice cream? The following steps will help you follow the food part of The
Loving Diet more easily.

1. Don't lose your sense of humor under any circumstances. As
   my dear friend told me once (and I swear I utter this quote least
   once a day), "You paid full price for this ticket." So while you
   are walking down the aisle at the grocery store, fill yourself
   with appreciation for how brave, amazing, and wonderful you
   are to have gotten to this very moment.

2. As best you can, stay in Phase 1 for six weeks. Keep in mind
   that you should be doing Phase 1 along with working with a
   practitioner, using supplements if warranted, examining your
   unique physiology, and following The Loving Diet exercises in
   Parts 1 and 2.

3. Try to loop in help from someone who will understand what you are doing. A nutritionist who specializes in Autoimmune Paleo, low FODMAP, and SIBO can help. A SIBO expert like Dr. Allison Siebecker (www.siboinfo.com) is essential. You can also visit my website www.aiplifestyle.com for a list of nutritionists who can work with you.

4. If you can't bring a nutritionist into the mix, just start where you are. Be open. Change what you eat. Take it day by day. Talk to a doctor who belongs to the Institute for Functional Medicine (IFM). Many times there are medical doctors covered by insurance who have specialized training and can help.

5. Eliminate all the health variables (maybe you have adrenal issues, anemia, or blood sugar problems and you don't know it?) before you start. Have comprehensive blood work or other tests done to find out (see Resources for more information). If you have a doctor who does not know how to do this, or does not believe in looking into your basic physiological function, use it as information for how you want to proceed.

6. Consider that you may need supplements to help heal your gut. I do not believe you can heal a leaky gut with diet alone. I cannot stress this enough. Diet alone is just a diet. Diet changes combined with all the supportive parts like supplements, loving, mindfulness, practitioner support, and uncovering physiology issues is a plan. Don't just follow the diet. Make yourself a plan! A properly trained practitioner will tell you what you will need to accomplish this. If you suspect you have SIBO, start there. Create a healing notebook and start taking notes of who you want to loop into your health-care plan and why. I also recommend anyone who has been trained by Datis Kharrazian DHSc, DC, MS, MNeuroSci (C), FAACP, DACBN, DABCN, DIBAK, CNS, as well as chiropractic neurologists from the Carrick Institute and doctors who practice functional medicine from the IFM. Try to find someone who has been trained about SIBO and autoimmune disease. Ask a lot of questions.

7. Gather your team. Seriously. Gather them. Your acupuncturist, your healer, your doctor, your nutritionist, your family, and your friends. Be ready to "fire" anyone who is not on board with your heart's desire for healing and how you will get there. Trust if you must find other care that it will come. And remember: Sometimes what appears as a stumble or fumble is actually a step forward because you uncover something meaningful about yourself. If it takes a few tries to get the *right* team, trust that.

8. If the food is not listed on the diet list, don't eat or drink it. I excluded the "do-not-eat" list from this book because it is so large. There are quite a few items that are allowed on the acceptable AIP list that I am asking you to remove. You can visit my website for a more detailed list of allowable and non-allowed AIP foods at www.aiplifestyle.com.

9. Know that this diet is not permanent; it is temporary. Soon enough you can move on to Phase 2 and Phase 3—eating a modified version of Autoimmune Paleo.

10. There is no real right or wrong. There is only what feels best to you. There are lots of diets out there to choose from. Many people have opinions. Those who say they know the right or wrong way always raise a big red flag for me. Ultimately we are all on the path to the same destination. I am offering you this path and I encourage you to use your heart to decide if it is right for you.

14

MY METHODOLOGY

You can do this.
I know you can.

♥

IN NUTRITION-SPEAK, THE FOOD portion of The Loving Diet is
AIP + SIBO + Low FODMAP together. In essence, this is a low-inflammatory diet that is low in bacteria, starches, sugars, and certain fibers. Let me explain.

As a full-time Autoimmune Paleo nutritionist, my days are filled with
talk about food, diet, and how to eat. There are several books that address the Autoimmune Paleo Diet, which was originally written about
by Loren Cordain, in his book *The Paleo Diet*. Other books include Robb
Wolf's *The Paleo Solution*, Diane Sanfilippo's *Practical Paleo* (my favorite
Paleo book), and Sarah Ballantyne's *The Paleo Approach*, which broadens
the definition of AIP eating. My book will only include the general outline of the established diet and its basic definition, since so many others
have wonderful resources for you to draw upon. I suggest you read all of
them. The goal of this book is to give you exactly what you need to get
started, encouragement to find a practitioner who can walk you through
healing the physiological aspects to your illness, and the tenants of The
Loving Diet in previous chapters to help you change the relationship you
have with your disease and life.

WHAT IS THE FOOD ELEMENT OF THE LOVING DIET?

The Autoimmune Paleo Diet is the Paleo Diet (no legumes, grains, dairy, sugar), but in addition, it eliminates:

- Nuts
- Seeds (including seed spices)
- Nightshades (tomatoes, all peppers, eggplant, tomatillos, and nightshade spices)
- Eggs

The Autoimmune Paleo Diet looks to reduce inflammation in the gut. That gut inflammation is a big driver of autoimmune disease. The diet also lowers the amount of inflammatory agents in our diet, namely lectins. (Again, I am very much simplifying the definition of AIP for the sake of this being a heart-mindfulness book and not a science book.)

Lectins are proteins that are difficult for the body to digest (commonly referred to as anti-nutrients) that are widespread in grains, nuts, and legumes. Nature designed lectins to survive nature, and that translates to our bodies not being able to digest them like other foods. Lectins cause changes both in immunity and physiology. Interestingly, lectins are also found in vegetables and many foods, but in lower levels. Lectins primarily cause IgM, IgG, and on occasion IgE antibodies. If a lectin protein binds to a specific carbohydrate at a cell, then the cell membrane is disrupted (cellular activities can also be disrupted), which can lead to autoimmunity. What this translates to in relation to the gut and digestion: Lectins may bind to enterocytes in the gut wall, causing lesions and inflammation, and the gut then becomes *leaky*. When this happens, it disrupts the production of enterokinase, which interferes with protein digestion and nitrogen absorption in the gut. So not only does the gut get leaky, but digestion is disrupted as well. The gut becomes leaky when the lectins bind to the gut wall, which loosens the tight junctions between the enterocytes and then increases intestinal permeability. This allows for both lectin and non-lectin proteins to pass through the gut wall into general circulation. Once through the gut wall, the lectins trigger the immune system to react to the disruption, so an immune response occurs. This can be a silent event happening over and over again in the gut—years on end for many people who have eaten grains for most of their lives.

I noticed, however, after counseling hundreds of clients on the Autoimmune Paleo Diet, that many people were not getting better as quickly as hoped. These clients were adhering to the diet perfectly, focusing on nutrient density and appearing quite dedicated. I knew there was more behind their complaints besides non-compliance that includes physiological factors like SIBO that were serious roadblocks to getting well. Getting this far in the book, it will also be obvious that in my opinion there are heart and soul issues related to illness that can be huge contributors to ill-health, too. Given that approach, however, I decided to create a more gut-focused diet that included the Autoimmune Paleo Diet, low FODMAP, and a SIBO diet. Because autoimmune disease has its roots in the gut, I created this modified Autoimmune Paleo Diet to offer a more comprehensive approach to gut issues. It has been estimated that one in five Americans have chronic bowel disease, so I decided to go hard and heavy and advance the Autoimmune Paleo Diet to address the gut microbiome in a more targeted program. It was only out of sheer frustration that I happened upon this combination of foods, and to my surprise, even the most difficult clients quite rapidly improved when I asked them to follow this diet.

It is known that a lot of AIPers need to be low FODMAP, but after an exhaustive trial and error with clients, I soon added resistant starch to the "do-not-eat" list, and The Loving Diet was complete. It is a rather limited diet, so I suggest working with a Loving Diet practitioner or a nutritionist who is well versed in Autoimmune Paleo, SIBO, and low FODMAP to help you transition to the diet. One important note: This diet is temporary, supplements are almost always needed, and depending on your body, the timing of how long you do each phase may vary. It will be a mixture of tracking inflammatory markers (the Cyrex Labs

Array 2: Intestinal Antigenic Permeability Screen as well as general inflammatory markers and antibody levels), keeping close tabs on your symptoms, and progressing toward good digestion.

THE MAIN GOALS OF THE LOVING DIET

My hope is that if you follow The Loving Diet, it will:

1. Reduce inflammation in your gut.
2. Support the basics of the Autoimmune Paleo Diet.
3. Change the populations of both SIBO and beneficial bacteria.
4. Reduce the amounts of sugar, starch, and fibers that feed SIBO, including resistant starch.
5. Lower the amount of fructans, fructose, and polyols that feed bacteria in gut by eating low FODMAP. (I do not include lactose in my definition of low FODMAP because AIP is a lactose-free diet.)

Again, The Loving Diet is meant to be a temporary diet, guided by a professional to make sure you are hitting all the macronutrient and micronutrient goals for your height and weight, given how limiting it is. Ideally, I recommend only eating Phase 1 for six to eight weeks under the care of a professional. You may also test positive for leaky gut or SIBO, and if you do, then in addition to this diet, you may need a complete gut-healing protocol. Gut-healing protocols have the following common goals in mind:

1. Kill or affectively reduce the populations of the bad bacteria by eating a low-bacteria diet, in addition to herbal and prescription SIBO antibiotics.
2. Heal the gut.
3. Grow populations of beneficial bacteria.

4. Lower inflammation.
5. Re-establish normal placement for bacterial populations from small intestine to large intestine.

I noticed in my client population that the Autoimmune Paleo Diet did not go far enough to heal the intestinal mucosa by itself, or in addition to healing protocols that attempted to do so in many cases. I see a lot of AIPers trying low FODMAP with some success. However, I am suggesting they go even further. My disclaimer here: Many folks feel great on AIP. This diet is not addressing those cases. I created this diet because the people who find me for help are not getting better on AIP alone. I also created this diet because there is a growing group who have autoimmune disease that are asking the big questions, such as, "How can I manage my suffering in this disease?" or "How can I find joy in the midst of disease?" or "How can my soul grow from my diagnosis?" My group goes beyond the traditional stress-reduction techniques and into the realm of soul searching. This diet, while limiting, is only part of your journey into your heart. Keep that in consideration as you read the list of allowable foods, and give yourself a little pep talk. The journey of your soul is greater than your diet.

PROFESSIONAL GUIDANCE

Tests can help determine the state of your gut, and working with an experienced professional can help you. If that's available to you, you might consider it. He or she may prescribe some gut function tests, such as the following:

1. Stool test that looks at digestion, parasites, and bacteria populations (Doctor's Data and Genova Diagnostics)
2. Cyrex Labs Array 2: Intestinal Antigenic Permeability Screen
3. SIBO breath test (Genova Diagnostics or Commonwealth Labs)
4. H. pylori test (breath, stool, blood)
5. Cyrex Labs Array 10: Multiple Food Immune Reactivity Screen

WHICH SPECIFIC SUPPLEMENTS CAN HELP HEAL THE GUT?

Once you are under the care of an experienced practitioner, you will want to work on rebuilding the gut bacteria populations. The following supplements can be beneficial:

1. SIBO-friendly probiotics and soil-based probiotics only
2. Herbal or prescription SIBO antibiotics like neomycin and rifaximin
3. Intestinal mucosa healers like L-glutamine
4. Butyrate supplements (due to the absence of resistant starch)
5. Brush border enzymes
6. Digestion supplements like betaine HCl and ox bile

Taking a SIBO-friendly probiotic (note: fermented foods and almost all probiotics are not SIBO-friendly) helps this process along. See the chapter below with reintroduction instructions for more information. An experienced practitioner may also include exercises that help with the motility of the gut, or address ileocecal valve issues. Vagus nerve stimulation through exercises is a brilliant way to increase gut motility. It can include diaphragm breathing, stimulating the gag reflex, gargling, and enemas. It is important, however, to address brain inflammation issues, as they often accompany gut issues. For that reason, I recommend chiropractic neurologists from the Carrick Institute to examine gut-brain issues.

CONTRIBUTORS TO GUT ISSUES

Other factors that could be contributing to gut dysbiosis besides your diet and leaky gut caused by the food you are eating include:

- Parasites
- Viruses
- Autoimmunity
- Dental infection
- Ulcers (H. pylori)
- Lack of digestive secretions
- Candida
- Food sensitivities
- Hypothyroid
- B-vitamin deficiencies
- MTHFR
- Brain inflammation
- Ileocecal-valve weakness
- Environmental toxin exposure
- Decreased gut motility
- Inflammation in the brain

WHAT IS THE LOVING DIET?

Paleo + Autoimmune Paleo + Low FODMAP + SIBO = The Loving Diet

LOW FODMAP DIET

Since I'm including the Low FODMAP Diet as part of The Loving Diet program, I will provide some background information about what this means. The Low FODMAP Diet was developed by Sue Shepherd and Peter Gibson from Monash University in Melbourne in 1999. It was originally developed for those suffering with IBS. FODMAP is the acronym for fermentable oligosaccharides, disaccharides, monosaccharides, and polyols. In simple terms, FODMAP foods break down into fructose in the intestinal mucosa and feed the less-desirable bacteria in the gut. These short-chain carbohydrates are not completely absorbed in the gastrointestinal tract and can be easily fermented by gut bacteria. The fermentation caused by these undigested sugars can cause IBS symptoms such as diarrhea, gas, and pain.

The Low FODMAP Diet removes foods that are high in:

- Oligosaccharides (fructans and galacto-oligosaccharides [GOS])
- Disaccharides (lactose)
- Monosaccharides (excess fructose)
- Polyols (sorbitol, mannitol, maltitol, xylitol and isomalt)

There are many common foods that are high in FODMAP that can potentially contribute to IBS symptoms, even if they are considered healthy by most standards. Lactose from dairy products; fructose from certain fruit, coconut products, and sweeteners; fructans from fibers in certain vegetables; and polyols from fruit and sugar alcohols are all rich in FODMAPs. It can be difficult for those with digestive issues or gut disorders to tolerate these foods. A high FODMAP diet can cause painful symptoms in those with IBS and Crohn's disease. Being intolerant to high FODMAP can bring on symptoms like gas, bloating, stomach pain, and indigestion.

I have modified numerous low FODMAP diets here to be autoimmune compliant. I have also taken into consideration the many low FODMAP lists floating around online. Many of you who are already well-versed in low FODMAP may see what you consider inconsistencies. In some cases, I choose to eliminate foods I typically see people react to on AIP (like coconut milk and coconut pulp) that are somewhat low FODMAP. Others, like starchy vegetables that seemed to have inconsistencies in portions, I occasionally rounded up for the sake of enough carbohydrates. I work with many, many women who do not do well on intermittent fasting or on a low-carbohydrate diet. Some do fine initially, others don't. It is a mixed bag, so use your own discernment and physiological markers to determine how low-carb you can go.

Personally, I cannot follow a low-carb regimen. If you see these discrepancies, note that my philosophy tends to "meet in the middle," and based on the kinds of issues I see clinically over and over again, I took them into consideration when formulating the diet. It was a process of about fifteen revisions until I found one that I felt was workable, considering that so many foods are already eliminated through the Autoimmune Paleo Diet. Also, I do not include a "do-not-eat" list. There are more foods you can't eat than you can, so I keep it simple. If the food is not listed on these pages, don't eat it.

A few important to things to remember about low FODMAP:

1. Cooking your vegetables may make them easier to digest.
2. It is best to individualize your diet as much as possible. You may not be sensitive to winter squashes, but even a small bit of avocado could bother you.
3. I recommend no more than 2 servings of the starchier vegetables each meal. See how you feel. If it bothers you, try 1 serving of starchier vegetables. If you are tired and dragging, you may need 3 servings of starchier vegetables per meal. There is no exact way.
4. The serving size listed in the chart is per meal. Some people eat four to five meals a day. That is okay.
5. Often fruit is best digested when eaten without other foods.

SIBO DIET

Since I incorporate the SIBO Diet into my plan, I will outline the basics. SIBO (small intestinal bacterial overgrowth) is gaining a lot of traction in the functional medical field. It is estimated that up to 80 percent of those with irritable bowel syndrome have SIBO. Overgrowth of certain bacteria in the small intestine can be problematic for many and result in symptoms of gas, bloating, constipation, and abdominal pain. SIBO is also notoriously difficult to treat and sometimes difficult to diagnose through common breath tests.

Bacterial overgrowth in the small intestine is due to a migration of native large intestine bacteria to the small intestine for various reasons. Low stomach acid, low intestinal motility, and a stressful lifestyle are some of the causes. Illness (IBS, H. pylori, and celiac, to name a few) and chronic constipation may weaken the ileocecal valve, contributing to the migration of the microbial environment from the large to small intestine. These "out-of-place" bacteria then feed on the not-yet-digested foods found in the small intestines, grow in numbers, and create a host of physical and digestive disturbances known as SIBO.

Because the large intestine inherently has a larger population of bacteria in comparison to the small intestine (almost ten times as many), bacteria normally found in the colon that takes up residence in the small intestine can cause profound changes. When this event takes place, the small intestine changes how well it can digest and absorb food, micronutrients, and amino acids. It in essence becomes more "leaky." When bacteria migrate from the large to small intestine, the bacteria are exposed to different foods in the form of starches, fibers, and sugars. These provide a rich source of food for the misplaced bacteria, which then grow in numbers in the small intestine. This creates the symptoms we now associate with SIBO. Furthermore, certain probiotics and fermented foods can aggravate this situation and add to the problem of overgrowth. Not because they are inherently bad, but because bacteria in the wrong place and at the wrong time grow in undesirable numbers, eating the probiotics and creating a gut problem. Functionally, when the small intestine environment is overgrown with bacteria, it cannot perform its normal functions of absorption, but SIBO can also create or exacerbate issues of leaky gut.

There is a way to help heal SIBO, although it can be a long and tricky path. Not all the treatments are effective, and some treatments need to be repeated. Working with a health-care practitioner is essential in this regard. Healing SIBO requires a few factors:

1. Diet: Low FODMAP (low fructose, no grains, no legumes)
2. Probiotics: SIBO-friendly blend only and some soil-based probiotics (this diet is essentially a low bacterial diet!)
3. Improving digestive secretions: Low pancreatic function or HCL production in stomach should be addressed. It will help with lowering bacterial populations in food and help increase brain-gut axis.
4. Increasing digestive motility: Working with a practitioner to design an individualized program
5. Gut healing supplement protocol
6. Antibiotics (pharmaceutical or herbal)
7. Prokinetic movements to strengthen and increase digestive motility

HOW TO TEST FOR SIBO

A breath test is the most up-to-date and widely available form of detecting SIBO. A sample of breath measures levels of hydrogen and methane. Different SIBO bacteria produce these gases in the small intestine. Breath tests for SIBO may not be as accurate as we would like. Although false positives are rarer, false negatives are common. It is best to work with a practitioner to assess symptoms and use that as a benchmark for treatment, along with a breath test. Because SIBO is so often found now in chronic digestive issues, I included it in The Loving Diet.

RESISTANT STARCH

A few words about resistant starch: Resistant starch is starch in food that's not absorbed in the small intestine by healthy people. It travels to the colon, where it is feasted upon by bacteria, which then produces short chain fatty acids that are extremely important for our immune system and colon health. Resistant starch is known to have many beneficial qualities like blood sugar regulation and the short chain fatty acids that are the primary fuel for colon cells. However, because my population has autoimmune disease, and there are some studies now that show rheumatoid arthritis, celiac, ankylosing spondylitis, and Crohn's disease can actually be worsened by resistant starch,[12] I have chosen to eliminate it from the first phases of The Loving Diet.

We know now that autoimmune disease can be related to bacterial populations in the gut. That the "wrong" populations of bacteria can crowd out the "right" populations (as in the case of SIBO), and dysbiosis can occur. A recent study showed that decreased bacterial diversity characterizes the altered gut microbiota in patients with psoriatic arthritis, resembling dysbiosis in inflammatory bowel disease. [13]

I opted to remove resistant starch from the diet, at least at first, then reintroduce it slowly after inflammation has reduced and symptoms have improved. While there is not a lot of resistant starch on AIP, it is allowed in the form of green plantains, bananas, taro, tapioca, and yucca root. I see those foods used quite often in AIP recipes and treats. I believe that many with autoimmune diseases suffer to some degree with adrenal gland issues. Reducing starch in the diet can be antagonistic in this regard with women especially, so I highly recommend keeping in moderate amounts of the allowable starches on this diet to maintain energy.[14] Note: Some people do very well with intermittent fasting. Some do extremely well phasing into ketosis. There are fantastic programs and practitioners out there that address these diets. I have quite a few clients who thrive on these diets. I am not discounting these routes, but for the sake of keeping things streamlined, I landed on keeping some carbohydrates in the diet, albeit limited amounts of carbohydrates, and the clinical results I see work for my clients in this diet. I just see women do better with moderate carbohydrate intake if they have autoimmune disease.

---

12 www.hindawi.com/journals/jir/2013/872632/.

13 http://onlinelibrary.wiley.com/doi/10.1002/art.38892/epdf.

14 www.ncbi.nlm.nih.gov/pmc/articles/PMC3678459.

RESISTANT STARCHES NOT ALLOWED DURING
PHASE 1 OF THE LOVING DIET:

- Green plantains
- Green bananas
- Green banana flour
- Green plantain flour
- Unripe bananas
- Cooked plantains
- Cassava starch (manioc, tapioca, yucca)
- White and lesser yam (note this is not sweet potato, although sweet potato is high FODMAP and not on the first phase of The Loving Diet)

My nutrition practice consists of those with autoimmune disease navigating their way through the Autoimmune Paleo Diet. Consistently, I see that there are gut issues that participate with autoimmune disease. And quickly I saw that the AIP diet was not enough, although many feel better when they are on it. So I reformulated the diet to be more comprehensive toward healing the gut by lowering starches, resistant starches, sugars, and fibers that contribute to leaky gut.

Why? Because most of my clients have leaky gut and other inflammatory gut issues. I thought, *Why not remove the triggers from the start?* So I looked at high FODMAP and resistant starch.

This kind of diet raises some very good questions floating around the Paleo community. Resistant starch has become extremely popular in the Paleo movement lately, due to helping regulate blood sugars, improve insulin sensitivity, and increase "good" colon bacteria populations.

That said, here is what I have found with my clients:

- They don't do well on a low-carbohydrate diet.
- Many have FODMAP sensitivity.
- They don't do well on resistant starches (at first).

- They have other gut issues like H. pylori (sometimes hernias!) or SIBO that are not being addressed.
- They can't find a practitioner to lead them through the low-carb phase, heal the gut, and remedy the factors contributing to the leaky gut.
- They need help navigating how to add resistant starch back into their diets after all aspects of gut dysfunction have been addressed.
- They tend to have some sort of brain-gut axis issue, like weak valves due to years of infections, low motility, or inflammatory bowel disease.

The need for a clinician to follow you on this journey is vital. He or she will assess/monitor the following:

- Butyrate levels from going low-carb
- Parasites
- SIBO
- Beneficial and pathogenic bacteria populations
- Leaky gut
- Intestinal IgA
- Food intolerances (I recommend Cyrex Labs Array 10)
- Inflammatory markers
- Digestive secretions affecting pH in gut, including brush border enzymes
- Blood sugar level/fasting glucose
- Adrenal/cortisol involvement
- Gut-brain axis issues

WHY AUTOIMMUNE PALEO ALONE MIGHT NOT BE ENOUGH

- There is a food in the AIP diet you might be sensitive to.
- Liver detoxification pathways are not robust enough (MTHRF gene mutations).
- Digestive function has not been restored.
- Inflammation has not been properly addressed.
- You have an infection that has not been diagnosed (like SIBO, virus, or dental infection).
- The brain-gut axis is impaired and has not been repaired.
- The hypothalamus-pituitary axis is impaired and has not been repaired.
- You have endocrine disruption in the form of hormone imbalance or adrenal dysfunction.
- The emotional/heart component of the autoimmunity has not been examined.
- There are micronutrient or macronutrient deficiencies.
- Blood sugar issues are present and are related to the entire endocrine system and brain function (even while on Paleo!).
- You have an undiagnosed anemia, hernias, bacterial or viral infections, or leaky valves.
- You are low FODMAP and resistant starch–intolerant.
- You have held beliefs that are not serving you any longer (like feeling you are not worthy).

A BIT MORE SCIENCE BEFORE YOU HIT THE GROCERY STORE

I'm not a medical doctor, so I cannot offer medical advice. The following is a discussion prompt for you with your doctor. He or she should know the answers. If not, find someone who does. Remember: You are at the edge of medicine. You are part of a medical revolution at this point. There are not a lot of medical practitioners practicing medicine that can address the whole of your issues. That is the good news and bad news. So, search for a practitioner with this in mind. If a doctor dismisses you and your symptoms, that is normal. He has reached the limit of how far he can heal you. Bless him and keep going. Keep listening to yourself and your heart. At the very least, these questions will get you and your doctor thinking!

If someone does not know how to look at lab work and food is the only piece being examined, it is only including part of the picture. If, for example, you see a moderately elevated MCV (mean corpuscular volume) on lab work, how would your practitioner proceed? When might she consider sending you to a doctor to rule out pernicious anemia? What if you have undiagnosed hemochromatosis and a well-meaning health coach strongly suggests adding organ meat to your diet? Would that be contraindicated? How would she tell the difference between moderate and mildly elevated liver enzyme markers? How do bio-identical hormones play a negative role in autoimmune disease? Are probiotics improving function or hindering it? How long should you be on digestive support? Why look at sodium markers on routine lab work? How can memory impairment be related to autoimmune disease and how can it be supported? What if you go on the Autoimmune Paleo Diet (like I did for a year) and you still have insulin-resistant hypoglycemia? Then what?

You can eat as much liver pâté and bone broth as you want, but if you are not improving function or absorption, then is it useful? Liver pâté may very well eliminate micronutrient lows, but does it matter if one is not addressing the impaired integrity of the intestinal mucosa? Does a low-inflammatory diet alone heal the intestinal mucosa? Does bone broth with natural levels of L-glutamine repair the intestinal mucosa? What is the role of adrenal glandulars and adrenal adaptogens? Do they go together? Should they be taken apart? What about the cytokine pathways? Are they relevant? What about the role of nitric oxide in your autoimmune disease? Should that be addressed? If you have a high homocysteine level, should you test for the MTHFR gene? Or just take methylated folate and B12? Do those even work? What if you have an autoimmune disease *and* an active viral infection (I see that one a lot)? What do you do then?

Above are just a sliver of the normal everyday issues I observe clinically with AIP clients. These are the extremely relevant concerns that can accompany the heart-mind-body challenges often at the root of autoimmune disease. These are critical questions to ask and critical questions that need to be addressed, in my opinion. You can't heal the thyroid without looking at the brain. You can't heal the brain without looking at inflammation. Autoimmunity is a truly multidisciplinary approach.

There are a multitude of factors that go along with health, healing, and The Loving Diet. Having a visionary approach not only helps you sort through the complexities of what you are facing but also helps to streamline the path to healing.

❤   ❤   ❤

Remember: Who is your team? What is their approach? How far are they willing to go to get you to where you need to go? There is a great divide in the healing world around autoimmunity. A number of practitioners are emerging who know about the Autoimmune Paleo Diet and how to support your efforts and physiology while on it. But how comprehensive is their approach?

If you have been doing the AIP diet and you are not feeling better, or as good as you hoped, there are still stones unturned. And if diet is the only component you are exploring, perhaps there is more that could be thoughtfully examined. There are still many, many options out there for you. Don't give up. The Loving Diet might just be your answer.

The most important thing I can say to you while you follow this diet is: Don't do it alone. Because along with the diet, I have clients selectively supplement to help support their particular situation. This can include getting rid of parasites or bacterial infections, rebuilding the immune system (if they have autoimmune disease and an active virus), SIBO-friendly probiotics, soil-based probiotics, butyrate supplements, and herbal and prescription SIBO antibiotics. If you try to *just follow the diet*, you may not be getting to the root of what is really going on, and your efforts may be in vain. It is worth finding a Datis Kharrazian–trained doctor or practitioner or a SIBO expert. Unfortunately, there are very few practitioners in the US who have a deep understanding of the low FODMAP/resistant starch/SIBO/AIP issue as a whole. I hope this will change soon. I came to this diet out of sheer frustration of so many clients not improving on AIP alone.

My bottom line: I love the Autoimmune Paleo Diet, but it does not do a good enough job healing the gut in many cases. When you get a good practitioner working with you, he will listen and test. Then he will listen and test again. It is easy to be dismissed by practitioners if you are in this category because you have traveled beyond the realm most practitioners have been trained for. That is good news, however. That is how the world changes. If enough people ask for more, eventually we hit a tipping point and medicine as we know it changes. You are asking yourself for more and you are asking health care for more. And when you do it from a loving place and not a victim place, you can travel quite far in the evolution of your heart.

I believe the practitioners out there who can offer help may do things like take a stool test and breath test and look at your adrenal glands, inflammatory markers, immune system, antibodies, leaky gut, any undiagnosed infections, and any dysregulated physiology like blood sugars or brain issues. It all works together. This diet is not easy. It is more challenging than the AIP diet. But it is the very best offering

I could assemble that really started making a dent for those who were not getting better. I am not opposed to starch or fiber. I just caution the use of them if you have other things going on, such as leaky gut or auto-immune disease. A skilled practitioner will help you sort through all of these issues. And if this is the first time you have ever read anything like this kind of approach, but you are nodding your head in agreement because something is resonating, don't give up.

15

GETTING STARTED

*The world is changing to meet you as a
result of coming into cooperation
with what ails you.*

♥

THERE ARE THREE PHASES to the food aspect of this diet:

- *Phase 1:* Elimination Phase
- *Phase 2:* Medium FODMAP Introductory Phase
- *Phase 3:* High FODMAP and Resistant Starch Introductory Phase

Find a notebook and keep a journal of everything you are eating and how you're feeling. This is extremely important so you can note what's not sitting right with you and what food might be bothering you as you introduce more.

HOW TO GROCERY SHOP

I suggest shopping twice per week to simplify your life. I don't like going to the grocery store more than twice a week so I suggest scheduling your shopping in that way. Make a list and get it done easily, but only twice. I prepare my meals for the week on Sundays because it is not a workday. I roast two cookie sheets of vegetables at once to save time, and I use parchment so I have limited cleanup. I also shop weekly deals at my grocery store and buy from local farmers. Because I eat a lot of greens and fresh vegetables, I shop twice a week. I use Instagram and Pinterest to plan my meals. I know you're busy and you have a lot of other things to deal with. Later in the book there are some recipes to get you started that are all phase-compliant.

One tip: When you buy greens or fresh herbs, wash them when you get home from the store and then wrap them in a clean, damp dish towel before storing them in the refrigerator. This will keep them from wilting.

- *Shop 1:* Days 1–4 food
- *Shop 2:* Days 4–7 food

WHAT DOES A LOVING DIET PLATE LOOK LIKE?

VEGETABLES: 50 PERCENT
FAT: 15 PERCENT
PROTEIN: 35 PERCENT

I usually use about one and a quarter pounds of protein. That provides about four servings—giving each person about 20 grams of protein each. I don't measure the fat, but I add a little more because it's a good anti-inflammatory food. If you're cooking for your family, you can still make a Loving Diet meal and make something additional on the side for them like rice or potatoes.

KEEP ON HAND AT ALL TIMES

There are certain foods that should always be in your home, because you will find yourself using them often. And you never want to leave yourself in a position where you are hungry and have nothing around that you are able to eat. Here are my suggestions for foods you may want to keep on hand:

- Bag of carrots
- Cooked pumpkin (frozen, fresh, organic canned)
- Cucumbers
- Cultured ghee
- Fresh/frozen fruit
- Frozen grass-fed beef
- Frozen chicken thighs
- Lemons
- Olive oil

PHASE 1

PHASE 1: HOW WILL YOU FEEL?

The first three days might be a little tough. You might:

- Be hungry
- Feel crappy
- Encounter sleep issues
- Feel tired
- Have headaches
- Have bowel changes

All of these are signs your body is readjusting to how you're eating. If these symptoms last for more than four or five days, talk to your practitioner.

After the first few days, you should have a decrease in bloating, your bowel movements should regulate, your digestion should improve, you should feel less puffy, and you should have more energy.

AIP/SIBO/Low FODMAP Protocol

FRUITS – LIMIT TO 2 SERVINGS PER DAY			
Avocado (1/8 avocado = 1 serving)	Honeydew Melon (1/2 cup)	Orange (1 orange)	Rhubarb (1 cup)
Cantaloupe (1/2 cup = 1 serving)	Kiwi (2 kiwis)	Papaya (1 cup)	Star fruit (1 star fruit)
Clementine (1 clementine = 1 serving)	Lemon	Passionfruit (1 passionfruit)	Strawberry (1/2 cup)
Dragonfruit (1 dragonfruit)	Lime	Pineapple (1 cup)	Tangelo (1 tangelo)
Grapes (1 cup)	Mandarin (2 mandarins)	Raspberry (1/2 cup)	Tangerine (1 tangerine)

VEGETABLES		
Arugula (limit to 1 cup per meal)	Chives (limit to 1/4 stalk per meal)	Olives (limit to 1/2 cup per meal)
Bamboo shoots (limit to 1/2 cup per meal)	Collard greens (limit to 1 cup per meal)	Parsnip (limit to 1/2 cup per meal)
Bok choy (limit to 1/2 cup per meal)	Cucumber (limit to 1/2 cup per meal)	Pumpkin (limit to 1/2 cup per meal)
Broccoli (limit to 1/2 cup per meal)	Endive (limit to 1/2 cup per meal)	Radish (limit to 6 radishes per meal)
Butternut squash (limit to 1/2 cup per meal)	Fennel (limit to 1/2 cup per meal)	Rutabaga (limit to 1/2 cup per meal)
Carrot (limit to 1/4 cup per meal)	Kale (limit to 1 cup, chopped per meal)	Spinach (limit to 1/2 cup per meal)
Celery Root (limit to 1/2 cup per meal)	Lettuce (limit to 1 cup, chopped per meal)	Swiss chard (limit to 1 cup per meal)
Celery (limit to 1/4 per serving)	Mustard Greens (limit to 1 cup, chopped per meal)	Turnip (limit to 1/2 cup per meal)
		Zucchini (limit to 1/2 cup per meal)

AIP/SIBO/Low FODMAP Protocol

PROTEIN	
Organic, grass-fed beef	Poultry
Fish	Shellfish
Organic, pasture-raised pork	

FATS		
Avocado oil	Duck fat	Olive oil
Bacon fat (from sugar-free, nitrate-free bacon)	Ghee, cultured	Red palm oil
Coconut oil	Lard	Tallow

HERBS	
Basil	Mint
Bay leaf	Oregano
Chives	Parsley
Cilantro	Rosemary
Cinnamon	Saffron
Edible Flowers	Sage
Ginger	Savory leaf
Lavender	Thyme
Lemongrass	Turmeric
Marjoram	Vanilla extract

PANTRY ITEMS	
Capers preserved in salt	Honey (limit to 1 tsp. per day)
	Maple syrup (limit to 1 tsp. per day)

DRINKS	
Mint tea	Ginger tea

PHASE 2

Follow Phase 2 for three to six weeks. As you enter Phase 2, you should not notice much difference. You will be tracking your bowel movements, digestion, and mental state. If you start to feel bloated, gassy, constipated, or foggy-brained, or have rashes, swelling, or aches, then stop, look at your food journal, and track back to what you ate and put on the *do-no-eat* list. Give yourself a day of Phase 1 eating and then start back in with the reintroductions.

PHASE 2
Reintroduce Medium FODMAP Foods

FRUITS – LIMIT TO 2 SERVINGS PER DAY							
Avocado (⅛ avocado = 1 serving)	Clementine (1 clementine)	Honeydew Melon (½ cup)	Lime	Papaya (1 cup)	Raspberry (1/2 cup)	Strawberry (1/2 cup)
Banana, unripe (1 banana)	Dragonfruit (1 dragonfruit)	Kiwi (2 kiwis)	Mandarin (2 mandarins)	Passionfruit (1 passion-fruit)	Rhubarb (1 cup)	Tangelo (1 tangelo)
Blueberries (1/2 cup)	Grapes (1 cup)	Lemon	Orange (1 orange)	Pineapple (1 cup)	Star fruit (1 star fruit)	Tangerine (1 tangerine)
Cantaloupe (1/2 cup)						

PROTEIN	
Organic, grass-fed beef	Shellfish
Bone broth	Organic, pasture-raised pork
Fish	Poultry

FATS		
Avocado oil	Duck fat	Olive oil
Bacon fat (from sugar-free, nitrate-free bacon)	Ghee, cultured	Red palm oil
Coconut oil	Lard	Tallow

Reintroduce Medium FODMAP Foods

VEGETABLES			
Arugula (limit to 1 cup per meal)	Carrot (limit to 1/4 cup per meal)	Kale (limit to 1 cup, chopped per meal)	Rutabaga (limit to 1/2 cup per meal)
Bamboo shoots (limit to 1/2 cup per meal	Celery Root (limit to 1/2 cup per meal)	Lettuce (limit to 1 cup, chopped per meal)	Sauerkraut (limit to 1 tsp. per meal)
Beets (1/2 cup per meal)	Celery (limit to 1/4 per meal)	Mushrooms (limit to 1 tbsp. per meal)	Spinach (limit to 1/2 cup per meal)
Bok Choy (limit to 1/2 cup per meal)	Chives (limit to 1/4 stalk per meal)	Mustard Greens (limit to 1 cup, chopped per meal)	Sweet potatoes (limit to 1/2 cup per meal)
Broccoli (limit to 1/2 cup per meal)	Collard greens (limit to 1 cup per meal)	Olives (limit to 1/2 cup per meal)	Swiss chard (limit to 1 cup per meal)
Brussel sprouts (limit to 1/2 cup per meal)	Cucumber (limit to 1/2 cup per meal)	Parsnip (limit to 1/2 cup per meal)	Turnip (limit to 1/2 cup per meal)
Butternut squash (limit to 1/2 cup per meal)	Endive (limit to 1/2 cup per meal)	Pumpkin (limit to 1/2 cup per meal)	Zucchini (limit to 1/2 cup per meal)
Carrot (limit to 1/4 cup per meal)	Fennel (limit to 1/2 cup per meal)	Radish (limit to 6 radishes per meal)	

PANTRY ITEMS		
Capers preserved in salt	Coconut milk OR Dried, unsweetened coconut (limit to 1/2 cup per day)	Honey (limit to 1 tsp. per day)
Coconut butter (limit to 1 Tbsp. per day)	Coconut sugar (limit to 1 tsp. per day)	Maple syrup (limit to 1 tsp. per day)

HERBS	
Basil	Mint
Bay leaf	Oregano
Chives	Parsley
Cilantro	Rosemary
Cinnamon	Saffron
Edible Flowers	Sage
Ginger	Savory leaf
Lavender	Thyme
Lemongrass	Turmeric
Marjoram	Vanilla extract

DRINKS	
Mint tea	Ginger tea

PHASE THREE

Spend three to six weeks reintroducing these foods. This phase will hopefully be where you stay, with the exception of any foods you are reacting to. See reintroduction protocol once you get started in this phase.

PHASE 3

Reintroduce High FODMAP Foods, Resistant Starch and Vinegars

FRUITS – LIMIT TO 2 SERVINGS PER DAY					
Apples	Blueberries	Kiwi	Orange	Pineapple	Strawberry
Apricots	Cantaloupe	Lemon	Papaya	Plantain, cooled	Tangelo
Avocado	Clementine	Lime	Passionfruit	Plum	Tangerine
Banana, ripe	Dragonfruit	Mandarin	Peach	Raspberry	Watermelon
Blackberries	Grapes	Mango	Pears	Rhubarb	
Cherries	Honeydew Melon	Nectarines	Persimmon	Star fruit	

PANTRY ITEMS	
Capers preserved in salt	Dried, coconut unsweetened
Coconut butter	Honey
Coconut milk	Fish sauce
Coconut sugar	Maple sugar
Coconut flour	Vinegars (apple cider, balsamic, red wine, white wine)

DRINKS	
Mint tea	Ginger tea

HERBS	
Basil	Mint
Bay leaf	Oregano
Chives	Parsley
Cilantro	Rosemary
Cinnamon	Saffron
Edible Flowers	Sage
Ginger	Savory leaf
Lavender	Thyme
Lemongrass	Turmeric
Marjoram	Vanilla extract

Reintroduce High FODMAP Foods, Resistant Starch and Vinegars

VEGETABLES			
Arugula	Cauliflower	Lettuce	Rutabaga
Artichoke	Celery Root	Leeks	Sauerkraut
Asparagus	Celery	Mushrooms	Shallot
Bamboo shoots	Chives	Mustard Greens	Radicchio
Beets	Collard greens	Okra	Spinach
Bok Choy	Cucumber	Onions	Sweet potatoes
Broccoli	Endive	Olives	Swiss chard
Brussel sprouts	Fennel	Parsley	Taro
Butternut squash	Garlic	Parsnip	Tigernuts
Carrot	Jerusalem Artichoke	Pumpkin	Turnip
Cabbage	Kale	Radish	Zucchini
			Yucca

FATS		
Avocado oil	Duck fat	Olive oil
Bacon fat (from sugar-free, nitrate-free bacon)	Ghee, cultured	Red palm oil
Coconut oil	Lard	Tallow

PROTEIN	
Bone broth	Poultry
Fish	Shellfish
Organic, grass-fed beef	Organic, pasture-raised pork

REINTRODUCTION OF HIGH FODMAP AND RESISTANT-STARCH FOODS

You will want to limit each of these foods to a serving. Follow what is typically a serving to you and your body, keeping in mind that a full cup of a starchy vegetable is usually a double serving.

- Artichoke
- Asparagus
- Avocado (whole)
- Cabbage
- Garlic
- Jerusalem artichoke
- Leeks
- Okra
- Onions
- Shallot
- Tiger nuts
- Apples
- Apricots
- Blackberries
- Cherries
- Dried fruits
- Fruit juices
- Grape

- Mango
- Nectarines
- Peach
- Pears
- Persimmon
- Plum
- Watermelon
- Plantain, cooled
- Taro
- Ripe banana
- Slow introduction of resistant starches (2 teaspoons/day): tapioca, manioc, yucca, yams, cassava, green plantains and bananas (and flour), and cooked plantains

BREAKFAST
(see recipes later in the book)

Sometimes breakfast can throw people for a loop, because they are so accustomed to eating grains or eggs. Keep it simple. Include a serving of a starchy carbohydrate (such as ½ cup of butternut squash) to regulate your blood sugar and support your brain. I usually eat the same kind of breakfast most days because it is easy. I like sausages and butternut squash with a tablespoon of cultured ghee. Don't skip it!

LUNCH

I tend to do two things for lunch: bring leftovers or make a big easy salad. I buy tubs of baby kale, spinach, and arugula. I keep grilled fish, chicken, and meatballs on hand in my refrigerator to assemble easy lunches. Carrots, radishes, and cucumbers on a salad with grilled fish is a lunch staple. Always keep a piece of fruit for yourself for an afternoon snack. I keep frozen soup stocked so that I can pull it out and heat it up if something shifts in my schedule and I need something quick. Get used to people commenting on how you eat or what you bring for lunch. Take it as a compliment, even if it sounds like it isn't. It's their issue, not yours.

RESTAURANTS

It is very hard to eat out at restaurants on this diet. It is helpful if you have an established relationship with a specific place because restaurants are notorious for taking great care of their regulars. Salads are a safe bet, but salad dressings almost never are. Bring your own dressing in a small jar. Order oven-roasted or grilled meats and seafood. Order foods that are as plain as possible, because sauces tend to have sugar or other added ingredients that you cannot have.

WHAT IF YOU'RE HUNGRY?

I allow two pieces of fruit a day with The Loving Diet. I suggest saving at least one of these servings for when you get hungry. Fat and protein also help us feel full. Use a dehydrator or use your oven on the lowest setting and make your own kale chips or zucchini chips (keep in mind kale is limited to 1 cup).

CAFFEINE

I suggest removing caffeine. It can perpetuate adrenal and cortisol issues, as well as blood sugar regulation. If you enjoy the ritual of your morning cup of coffee, try switching to mint or ginger tea.

ALCOHOL

Alcohol is a known contributor to SIBO. It can weaken valves and slow motility. I suggest taking a break from alcohol while doing The Loving Diet program.[15, 16] You can try reintroducing it in small amounts when you have finished. In the meantime, if you want to enjoy "happy hour" with friends or family, try pouring sparkling water in a wine glass. It will feel like a splurge.

BACON

Bacon is allowed on this diet, but it must be nitrate and sugar free. You will almost always have to order this online, find it at Whole Foods, or search it out at your local grocery store. It does exist. Places like US Wellness Meats carry it.[17]

---

15 www.ncbi.nlm.nih.gov/pubmed/25062877.
16 www.ncbi.nlm.nih.gov/pubmed/8447153.
17 http://grasslandbeef.com/.

PESTICIDES, PRESERVATIVES, AND ENVIRONMENTAL TOXINS

The reason The Loving Diet suggests that you make all of your food yourself and buy organic is to ensure you're not finding any of these extra ingredients on your plate. Preservatives, pesticides, and environmental toxins are chemicals, and every chemical we put into our body requires the liver to break it down. We also know now that there is a very real possibility you could be producing antibodies to these chemicals. Cyrex Labs Array 11 tests for mold, heavy metals, and environmental pollutants, in case you are interested in finding out if there is a connection for you.

Pesticides are being implicated in some autoimmune diseases like lupus and rheumatoid arthritis.[18, 19] Therefore, I suggest you know the sources of your foods, stay away from plastic, non-organic food, and avoid preservatives. I also very much caution against chelation therapy if you have autoimmune disease and think you may have heavy metals. If you have antibodies to metals and attempt to chelate them, you could be fueling the autoimmune fire and ultimately become sicker than before you started.

The chemicals found in processed foods, for example, run counter to The Loving Diet. Having said that, in keeping with the spirit of the diet, don't become polarized against them—don't have a strong opinion of them. Just avoid them. Genetically modified foods (GMOs) are something I do not ever buy. But they're not the enemy. Our thinking that they are the enemy is the enemy. When you become polarized about what is good and bad, it sets us up for againstness, and the health I am looking for is not found in againstness. I do not eat GMOs, nor do I recommend them. But I also don't put a lot of thought into them. I put thought into what is working for me and how to get there. They're like the illness: They're a player giving us information to help us choose

18 http://nihrecord.nih.gov/newsletters/2011/03_18_2011/story4.htm.
19 www.rodalenews.com/natural-insecticide.

ourselves. I'd say don't choose them, but don't create againstness by hating them. Instead:

- Prepare your own food.
- Buy natural ingredients and support local farms.
- Check the organic sections at even the big grocery chains and also buy online.
- Read labels.
- If you're tight on time, do the best you can.

SUPPLEMENTS FOR *ALL* PHASES

The following supplements can be taken during Phase 1, Phase 2, and Phase 3. It's best to consult a practitioner for use.

- Prescript-Assist (SIBO-friendly bacteria, Lactobacillus casei, Bifidobacterium breve, and Lactobacillus plantarum, and soil probiotics)
- Betaine HCL with ox bile
- Ox bile or pancreatin
- L-glutamine
- Vitamin D3
- SIBO antimicrobials and/or prescription
- Brush border enzymes
- Essential fatty acids
- Liposomal curcumin (turmeric)
- Butyrate (to take the place of reduced amounts of resistant starch)—titrate off butyrate in Phase 2 and remove in Phase 3 due to the reintroduction of resistant starch

Note: This is a general list of supplements. It's best to work with a practitioner who is well versed in assisting you to create your own plan of supplements and help with proper dosage.

16

FOOD REINTRODUCTIONS

Food is not the enemy,
but the resistance to change can be.

♥

FOOD REINTRODUCTIONS ARE AN intuitive process, but everyone wants them to be straightforward. Sorry to burst the bubble. Because I see so many clients who reintroduce foods after being on this diet, I am going to tell you that food reintroductions sometimes don't work, add up, or make sense. For instance, I added almonds back into my diet and I was fine for five months on them. Then I ate them a bit too frequently and I started having horrible stomach pains and gas. I have not been able to add them back into my diet even though I was once fine with them. Food reintroductions are considered the gold standard, but doing so can be tricky. It's not a perfect science, so go in knowing that. Size and frequency matter when you are reintroducing foods. If you eat a food too often or have too much of it, there is a chance you may start reacting to it *even if you never have before.* I never in my life had an issue with almonds before I started reacting to them. Go figure. Food is weird. Bodies are weird. It's just the way it is. So when you read on, don't get hung up on the details if it doesn't go the way you plan or think. Get Zen about it.

The following steps will help you navigate your food reintroductions more easily:

1. Keep a food journal and don't forget to use it.
2. Introduce one food every five days. When you introduce a food in that five-day period, try the following:
   - *Day 1*: Eat 1 teaspoon of the food at breakfast, 1 tablespoon of the food at lunch, and a small serving of the food at dinner. *If at any time you notice a reaction, immediately stop the introduction.*
   - *Day 2*: Eat another serving of the food at breakfast then stop eating the food.
   - *Days 3–5*: Wait three days and just watch to see how you feel.
3. There are two kinds of symptoms that accompany a food reaction. Physical and mental. Be on the lookout for these symptoms. Common physical symptoms include:
   - Headache
   - Rashes
   - Mucous
   - Muscle aches
   - Joint aches
   - Acne
   - Stomachaches
   - Gas
   - Bloating
   - Vision disturbances
   - Nausea
   - Racing heartbeat
4. Common mental symptoms include:
   - Lethargy
   - Brain fog
   - Depression
   - Anxiety
   - Vertigo
   - Lack of concentration
   - Crying or feeling emotional
   - Anger
   - Sadness
5. It can take up to seventy-two hours for a food sensitivity reaction to occur. The reaction can be physical or mental.
6. If you have a food reaction, wait three days to reintroduce another food.

17

LOVE THE FOOD

Food has a tremendous
power of healing.

♥

WHEN WE LOVE OUR food, we're automatically putting ourselves in a state of cooperation. It's what we're thinking before we start eating it. Generally, we're polarized around food. Food is both the enemy and the healer, due to how we've categorized it. It can be inflammatory. It can be GMO. It can have pesticides. It can be overly processed. It can be non-nutrient dense. Those lines divide us and make the food work against us. At the same time, food is extremely important. Food can work *for* us when we eat it and it reverses micronutrient deficiencies. It can reduce inflammation in the intestinal mucosa. It can provide us with the essential macronutrients for metabolism. It can make us feel good. It can feed the good bacteria in the upper small intestines and the lower intestines that can help us make neurotransmitters to make our brains work the right way. If people take the perspective that before they start eating, they love their food, then that can translate into deeper healing inside the body.

HOW TO LOVE THE FOOD

Put your food on your plate. Take a moment, either thanking it or telling it you love it—or even both.

NEVER SAY NEVER

You are only human. Even though I'm asking you to make an effort to stick to The Loving Diet protocol, remember that even if you slip, you're never off the path. Slip, and get back up and keep trying. There is a large amount of wisdom that can be fostered by loving yourself while you are slipping up. That's all you can do. I believe in you. I believe you can do this and I believe you have the tools. To help prevent slipping, grab a pad of Post-its. Write yourself a bunch of notes that read:

- I got this!
- This is good for me.
- This is happening to help me.
- I can do this.

Now post those stickies all over you house: inside the fridge, inside the cupboards, on your bathroom mirror—places you can see when you're brushing your teeth or getting food. When you see the note, appreciate your willingness to do something different. It isn't easy, and that's okay. If it feels hard and you mess up, that's okay. But use the notes to help you and keep you going. And get up each day and continue to try.

GETTING STARTED / FAMILY

My guess is that since you've been suffering already, it won't be too difficult to get motivated to do something different. Most of my clients find me when they're desperate, frustrated, or are seriously ready for something profound to touch their lives that hasn't yet. With a lot of diets, people with families struggle to make separate meals, and the planning and timing of cooking becomes challenging. With The Loving Diet, it's not so difficult. You cook the protein and veggies for everyone—your spouse and your kids—and you cook them an additional starch. I also do much of my weekly cooking on Sundays. I roast pans of veggies, tear up the greens, and shop for all of my protein. And my One-Pot Paleo meals, which you can find in chapter nineteen, will be time-saving as well.

❤   ❤   ❤

Remember, with any of this: We're not striving for perfection. We're striving for loving. If you eat something that doesn't sit well—maybe you learn preservatives don't settle well in your system—be happy you discovered some great information from that. That will arm you with new ways to take care of yourself in a different way.

And while eating in a way that might at first feel limiting, love what is in front of you. Walk up and down the aisle of the grocery store and see what jumps out at you. You might discover that a new locally grown vegetable is delicious. Just go into your grocery store or to your local farmers' market with openness and love—in cooperation instead of the opposite. Your openness will lead you to cool things, whatever they may be. Who knows what will inspire you when you're open to it in your life. Let it all work for you, not against you. Instead of hating the diet, love it, and the joy of it will come to you more easily. If you embrace it and have some fun trying new recipes, you will change your focus from feeling deprived to feeling excited that you now have some delicious new recipes in your repertoire.

When I'm in the grocery store, I do this a lot. I'll pick up food and think, *Look at how great I'm taking care of myself right now. I love grocery shopping, and I love picking out fresh oranges.* I do this when cooking, too.

*M*y client Stephanie was initially deeply disturbed not to have cereal or English muffins for breakfast when she started The Loving Diet for her hypothyroidism. But she started putting love into making her frisée salad with pancetta and actually being excited she had the time and luxury of eating one of her favorite French dishes every day for breakfast. She began putting the same love into her eating and found suddenly, for the *first time in a lifetime of being a professional dieter, that she came at the food from a place of luxe, not lack. Instead of focusing on everything she could not have, she spent the time enjoying and loving all the stuff she suddenly could have. She felt zero depriva-tion.* Her friend even texted her, Are you at least going to have some chocolate on Valentine's Day? *She responded,* No, in-stead I'm having my endive salad and loving myself. *Rather than eat a cupcake instead of having a date, she was going to love herself. Previously she would have considered this a crazy notion. One other note: She simply does the best she can do. She likes wine, so sometimes she will allow herself a glass. On occasion, she needs a pre-workout option, so she will have an almond en-ergy bar, once a week. She doesn't freak out like the sky is falling. She doesn't get angry at herself. She just enjoys and loves what she can do and accepts what she can't. A big progression from the win-fail mentality that was the basis of her eating for so many years in her life.*

18

NUTRIENT DENSITY

Attention follows intention.

♥

NUTRIENT-DENSE FOODS ARE FOODS that contain higher amounts of micronutrients per serving than other foods. We see that when people enter into the disease state, there's usually silent inflammation that we want to reduce through a low-inflammatory diet. There's also a nutrient-dense diet that we want to put people on, which will help course-correct micronutrient deficiencies. When we're stressed outwardly and we know we feel stressed, we use micronutrients for the body to help handle itself. Its micronutrient demands increase to help us deal with the stress. When we have silent inflammation, the same thing occurs. The body tries to correct itself. So it does this physiologically, through using micronutrients, to help heal itself. When we go on a nutrient-dense diet, we are increasing our micronutrient load in each meal. Since micronutrient deficiencies are connected to disease, it is an extremely important consideration. For the sake of course-correcting gut issues, however, I am leading with the gut-healing properties of this diet and embracing nutrient density as the backdrop for eating in general as you make your way through your life.

NUTRIENT-DENSE FOODS

- Broccoli
- Grass-fed meats
- Greens
- Leafy vegetables
- Liver / organ meats
- Root vegetables

HIGH-INFLAMMATORY FOODS

Vegetable oils (sunflower, safflower, canola, soy, cottonseed)
Omega-6 vegetable oils
Grains

PSEUDO-GRAIN WATCH LIST

Quinoa has received a lot of buzz lately because of its protein value. It is considered a pseudo-seed, or some people call it a pseudo-grain. That makes it a gray area in my book and also not AIP-compliant. I tell my autoimmune clients that if they want to get tested and find out if they are sensitive to quinoa, they can do a gluten cross-reactivity test when they first start AIP. It tests proteins in foods that are not from gluten but sometimes can act like gluten. So they're cross-reactive. The body thinks it's getting gluten, but it's not. That Cyrex test has foods that are potential cross-reactors to gluten that are common in gluten-free foods like quinoa. Tapioca is another one, and it's in many gluten-free foods as well as AIP recipes and treats I see online and in cookbooks. It's a starch that acts as a natural emulsifier or binder that is also eliminated in Phase 1 of The Loving Diet due to it having higher levels of resistant starch but also because it can be a potential gluten cross-reactor.

AIP ISN'T SYNONYMOUS WITH GLUTEN-FREE

When people follow a gluten-free regimen, they trade one grain for another, and that can continue to damage the intestinal mucosa, because grains, inherently, are inflammatory in nature. So rice, for example, does not contain gluten, but rice is a high-gluten cross-reactivity food. Rice bread is a popular gluten-free bread alternative. Not everyone reacts to it, but they can, and it's for two reasons. One is that rice can be a gluten cross-reactor, but another is that rice can also raise blood sugars quickly. Unstable blood sugars are a big source of inflammation in people's bodies.

There's a big difference here: Everyone thinks that maybe they can't eat gluten because they have celiac disease. Celiac disease is a hypersensitivity to even minute amounts of gluten. It's an autoimmune disease, and it's very clear-cut, but what we're finding now is that there's this whole movement inside the gluten-free movement, which is called gluten sensitivity. It is a sensitivity to gluten that produces antibodies, but it's not an autoimmune disease, and it's not a hypersensitivity to gluten. Doctors are having a hard time recognizing and looking for it and being able to properly test. Most doctors only test for three antibodies to gluten, if they perform a gluten test. There are more like twenty-four or twenty-five to be tested, as they pertain to gluten and they all don't point to celiac, but rather to gluten sensitivity. There's a whole movement that's beginning to change the idea of what determines gluten sensitivity.

VEGETARIAN VERSUS AIP AND PALEO PROTOCOL

One of the top questions I get asked about in regard to AIP and The Loving Diet is, "If I am a vegetarian, can I do it?"

The short answer to this is, "No."

But let me give a long answer, too. I have had some life-long vegetarians go on a six-week AIP program. All of them started eating animal protein in some form. Because the diet is so specific in its scope, it is critical to get plenty of protein. Protein is important for repairing the immune system and helping with the liver detoxification pathways. Protein (as a macronutrient) can also help with unstable blood sugars and collagen building.

So my vegetarian clients did a few things to help with the transition. They ate no (or very little) red meat and chose instead turkey, fish, and chicken. And, more important, they took digestive enzymes that increase acidity in the stomach. There is no hard science that I have found that connects vegetarians' digestive secretions changing over time on a vegetable diet, but there is plenty of anecdotal evidence in the professional world that this is the case. And I have seen many times that when vegetarians give themselves extra digestive support, their adverse reactions to meat decrease, and in some cases they actually start craving meat. Perhaps there was an aversion over time to eating meat purely because the body was guiding cravings in part from a lack of enzymes to digest the very food they were avoiding. The body adapting to its environment is a common physiological process, so I assume it can happen in these cases as well.

The very nature of vegetarianism from a micro level is what works against those with an autoimmune disease and yet gets the gold standard approval from sources such as the Mayo Clinic, who recommend 6–8 servings of whole grains a day to lower risk for heart disease and cancer. Lurking in every serving of grains and legumes (and all foods in varying amounts), however, are lectins.

EXERCISE

Exercise in whatever way feels right. You're not reading this to lose weight; you're reading this to improve your relationship with your disease.

Moving your body is important. Depending on the physical limitations, due to your disease, you can move through yoga, Pilates, walking, or whatever you enjoy. I like CrossFit, but that's my personal preference. Whatever you choose, moving is important. It increases circulation to the brain, which is crucial for autoimmune disease. Whatever you do, however, check in with your health-care professional first. Don't start anything new until you get clearance.

Take brisk walks. Don't overdo it: Over-exercising causes againstness, because in some people, it releases hormones in their brains that they're addicted to exercise. Over-exercisers need to exercise less.

People exercise differently. Some hypothyroid women want to eat fewer calories; some people feel that when they switch over to this diet they actually need to eat more, because they don't ever feel full. It's an individual thing that you should work on with a health-care practitioner to find out what your calories in should be, if you're interested in that. I never, ever ask my clients to count calories. Ever. If people saw how much fat I ate, it would probably shock them. Peace, joy, and love in life is job one. Inflammation-reduction is job two.

19

RECIPES

The best place to start your meal
is in a place of appreciation.

❤

WHEN I COOK AT home, like many of you, I'm often in a rush. I'm working, I'm raising a daughter, and I'm trying to cram a lot in. I started trying to do two things: prepare as much as I can on Sundays and make everything in one dish for dinner whenever I can. It started with something quick: stuffing ground lamb into squash halves, surrounding them in the pan with other veggies, and pouring olive oil on top. Occasionally, I would post a picture of that one-dish wonder on Instagram or Facebook. I was amazed by the interest those recipes generated! More amazing, I fed my family with about twenty minutes of my sweat. The rest was baking time. Brilliant!

In the later phases, you might be able to do more one-dish Paleo cooking, which is fast and easy. You simply put protein, veggies, and fat into a baking dish and bake it all together. But in Phase 1, it's too challenging based on the limits. On the following pages, you will find recipes for breakfast, lunch, and main courses.

BENEFITS OF ONE-DISH PALEO FOR PHASE 3

- Efficient
- Nutrient-dense
- Guarantees food is made from scratch
- Streamlined prep
- Hits all the points a meal needs: vegetables, starch, and protein

ANTI-INFLAMMATORY FATS

- Olive oil
- Coconut oil
- Lard
- Palm oil
- Bacon grease
- Cultured ghee

PARSNIP LEMON HASH WITH ROSEMARY PORK SAUSAGES

MAKES 4 SERVINGS

1 teaspoon smoked sea salt

2 tablespoons chopped lemon

2 tablespoons chopped fresh rosemary

1 pound ground pasture pork

1 tablespoon coconut oil

2 cups chopped parsnips

1. In a bowl, mix smoked salt, lemon, rosemary, and ground pork.
2. Form into 2-inch patties.
3. In a skillet, heat coconut oil and cook patties until cooked through, about 8 minutes.
4. Remove from pan, leaving drippings behind.
5. Peel skin off of parsnip. Dice into 1-inch pieces and add to skillet. Cook covered on medium until tender, about 15 minutes, stirring occasionally.
6. Serve with cooked patties.

BUTTERNUT PORRIDGE WITH CINNAMON AND BACON

MAKES 4 SERVINGS

8 slices bacon (nitrate and sugar free)

1 heaping cup chopped, skinned, and seeded butternut squash

2 teaspoons cinnamon

1. Preheat oven to 350°F.
2. Place bacon on a rimmed cookie sheet. Bake in oven for 20 minutes or until brown and crispy. Set aside bacon.
3. Reserve 1 tablespoon of bacon fat (put the rest in a mason jar and keep in fridge for future use).
4. Steam butternut squash until tender, about 15 minutes.
5. In a bowl, smash squash with a fork and add 1 teaspoon of extra bacon fat and cinnamon. Blend with fork. Top each serving with 2 pieces of crumbled bacon.

PUMPKIN WITH AVOCADO AND CULTURED GHEE

MAKES 4 SERVINGS

1 cup pumpkin puree

2 tablespoons cultured ghee

Salt to taste

1 teaspoon fresh grated ginger

1/2 avocado

1. Heat pumpkin puree with cultured ghee on medium heat in saucepan (I use organic canned pumpkin, frozen pumpkin, or pumpkin in my freezer from winter).

2. Add pinch of salt and fresh grated ginger. Heat for 5 minutes. Remove from heat and set aside.

3. Slice avocado and dice into 1-inch pieces. Divide into four servings and garnish pumpkin with avocado.

BREAKFAST SAUSAGES WITH GINGER AND KALE

MAKES 2 SERVINGS (10 SAUSAGES)

2 cups baby kale

2 pounds grass-fed beef

1 teaspoon salt

2 teaspoons fresh grated ginger

1. Preheat oven to 350°F.
2. In a food processor, blend kale, beef, salt, and ginger just until blended.
3. Form into 3-inch patties and bake on cookie sheet in oven for 25 minutes.

ZUCCHINI PORK PARSLEY SAUSAGES

MAKES 2 SERVINGS

11/2 cups shredded zucchini
1 teaspoon salt
1 pound ground pasture pork
1/2 cup parsley

1. Preheat oven to 350°F.
2. In a food processor, blend all the ingredients just until mixed.
3. Form into 3-inch patties and bake on cookie sheet in oven for 25 minutes.

SALAD DRESSINGS

MAKES ONE JAR

RASPBERRY LIME

1/2 cup fresh or frozen raspberries
2 tablespoons lime juice
1/2 cup olive oil
Pinch of salt

1. Macerate raspberries with a fork. Press through a sieve or strainer to remove seeds.
2. In a small bowl, whisk raspberries with lime juice, olive oil, and salt.

TARRAGON DRESSING

2 tablespoons fresh chopped tarragon
1/2 cup olive oil
Pinch of salt
2 tablespoons fresh lemon juice

Whisk all ingredients with a fork and store in a mason jar.

SIMPLE LEMON DRESSING

2 tablespoons fresh lemon juice

1 teaspoon honey

Pinch of salt

1/2 cup olive oil

Whisk all ingredients with a fork and store in a mason jar.

BASIL DRESSING

1 cup fresh basil

3/4 cup olive oil

2 tablespoons lemon juice

Pinch of salt

Blend all ingredients in a food processor until smooth. Store in the fridge.

ARUGULA, CUCUMBER, AND CARROT SALAD

MAKES 4 SERVINGS

4 medium shredded carrots

1 medium skinned and seeded cucumber

Olive oil

4 cups baby arugula

Tarragon dressing

1. Toss carrots and cucumber together with olive oil.
2. Toss in arugula and add 1 tablespoon tarragon dressing and toss again.

SHAVED FENNEL AND RADISH SALAD WITH SHRIMP

MAKES 4 SERVINGS

12 medium unpeeled shrimp

1 head fennel

1 orange

Pinch of salt

1 tablespoon olive oil

2 cups radishes

1. Preheat oven to 375°F.
2. Bake shrimp on a cookie sheet for 10 minutes.
3. On a cutting board with a sharp knife, core out the center of the fennel and any outer tough pieces. As thin as you can, cut the fennel root. Measure out 2 cups of fennel and place in bowl.
4. Zest orange over bowl and add salt and olive oil.
5. Chop radishes into 1-inch pieces and toss with fennel.
6. Remove shrimp from oven and let cool. Remove shells and arrange 4 shrimp on top of each salad.

PORK CHOPS WITH CELERY ROOT AND CARROT-RADISH SALAD

MAKES 4 SERVINGS

1 cup grated carrots

1 cup grated radishes

1 cup chopped and skinned cucumber

2 teaspoons olive oil

2 teaspoons chopped oregano

$1/2$ teaspoon salt

1 cup chopped and skinned celery root

1 tablespoon cultured ghee, divided

4 pasture pork chops

1. Preheat oven to 375°F.
2. Grate carrots and radishes.
3. Cut cucumber into 1-inch pieces. Toss in olive oil, oregano, and pinch of salt. Set aside.
4. Cut celery root into 1-inch pieces. Steam until tender. Mash with fork and add pinch of salt. Add 1 tablespoon of ghee and mix.
5. Place pork chops on cookie sheet. Sprinkle each with a pinch of salt. Oven-roast until they reach an internal temperature of 145°F. Remove from oven and let rest for 3 minutes.
6. To plate, scoop mashed celery root onto each plate. Place pork chop on top and then top each with a serving of the carrot-radish salad.

PORK LOIN STUFFED WITH SPINACH AND SAGE

MAKES 4 SERVINGS

2 cups baby spinach

2 teaspoons olive oil

1 pasture pork loin (they are usually around 2 pounds)

1–2 teaspoons salt

18 fresh sage leaves

1 bunch fresh chives

1. Preheat oven to 375°F.
2. Quickly sauté baby spinach with olive oil just until wilted.
3. Open the loin with your fingers or slice an opening down the middle to open it up if it is not pre-sliced. Sprinkle inside of pork loin with a few pinches of salt.
4. Arrange sage leaves long ways across loin. Place chives long ways as well. Evenly spread spinach in loin and using butcher twine and toothpicks, tie up the loin.
5. Roast in oven until pork reaches internal temperature of 145°F. Let sit for 3 minutes after removing from oven and slice to serve.

BEST GREEN CHICKEN THIGHS

MAKES 4 SERVINGS

1 cup fresh basil leaves

1 cup fresh cilantro leaves

1/2 cup olive oil

1/2 zucchini

1 tablespoon fresh lemon juice

2 teaspoons salt

2 pounds chicken thighs (bone in, skin on)

1. Preheat oven to 375°F.
2. Blend basil, cilantro, olive oil, zucchini, lemon juice, and a pinch of salt in blender until smooth to make green sauce.
3. In an oven-safe baking dish, arrange chicken thighs. Pour green sauce over the chicken and bake uncovered for 45 minutes. Turn heat down if it seems to be burning (check about 30 minutes into cooking for this).

HALIBUT WITH SAFFRON AND MASHED TURNIPS

MAKES 4 SERVINGS

4 cups diced and peeled turnips

Pinch of salt

Zest from 1 lemon

5 teaspoons cultured ghee, divided

1 pinch saffron

4 (8-ounce) pieces of halibut

1. Steam turnips until tender. Mash and add salt, lemon zest, and 3 teaspoons cultured ghee. Set aside.
2. In a skillet pan, heat 2 teaspoons cultured ghee and add saffron. Add halibut (you will need to do this in batches) and cook for 4–5 minutes each side.
3. Serve halibut over mashed turnips.*

I usually add a few handfuls of fresh baby spinach or arugula on top of the halibut.

SCALLOPS WITH CAPERS AND PARSNIPS

MAKES 4 SERVINGS

2 cups peeled and diced parsnips

1 tablespoon olive oil

Salt to taste

2 tablespoons cultured ghee, divided

12 medium-sized scallops

1/4 cup chopped chives

1/4 cup salted capers

1/4 cup unpeeled, diced, fresh lemon

1. Preheat oven to 375°F.
2. Dice parsnips into 2-inch pieces. Toss with olive oil and salt and roast in oven, on a parchment-lined cookie sheet, for 30 minutes.
3. In a skillet, heat 1 tablespoon ghee on medium-high heat. Working in two batches, place scallops in skillet after ghee is heated. Cook 3 minutes each side.
4. Remove parsnips from oven. Place in bowl and toss with 1 tablespoon ghee, lemon, capers, and chives. Serve with scallops.

ALL-PURPOSE MEATBALLS WITH GREENS

MAKES 4 SERVINGS

2 teaspoons sea salt, divided

2 pounds grass-fed beef

1 tablespoon chopped fresh thyme

1 tablespoon chopped fresh rosemary

1 tablespoon chopped fresh oregano

2 cups spinach

2 tablespoons cultured ghee

1 pound chard (stems removed)

1. Preheat oven to 350°F.
2. In a food processor, blend 1 teaspoon smoked salt, beef, herbs, and spinach until mixed. Form into 2-inch meatballs. Bake on rimmed cookie sheet for 25 minutes.
3. In a large cast-iron skillet or sauté pan, add ghee. Tear chard into pieces with your clean hands and add to skillet. Sauté until wilted, about 4–5 minutes. Sprinkle with 1 teaspoon smoked salt.
4. Serve meatballs atop sautéed chard.

BROCCOLI MEATLOAF

MAKES 4 SERVINGS

1 cup broccoli florets

1 cup shredded carrots

Zest of 1 lemon

1 teaspoon salt

1 1/2 pounds ground organic turkey

1. Preheat oven to 350°F.
2. In a food processor, blend broccoli and carrots. Add lemon zest, salt, and turkey and blend until mixed.
3. Form into a loaf and bake on a parchment-lined, rimmed cookie sheet for 45 minutes.
4. Serve while warm.

CHICKEN BREAST STUFFED WITH SAGE OVER BOK CHOY AND FENNEL

MAKES 2 SERVINGS

1 cup fennel root

4 heads bok choy

1 tablespoon olive oil

2 organic chicken breasts (bone in and skin on)

6 sage leaves

Salt to taste

1 tablespoon fresh thyme

1. Preheat oven to 350°F.
2. With a paring knife, core out the dense center portion of fennel root and discard. Slice remaining root as thinly as possible. Measure out 1 cup and set aside.
3. Rough chop bok choy. In a cast-iron skillet, add olive oil, fennel, and bok choy. Sauté until bok choy starts to soften, about 8 minutes. Remove from heat.
4. Carefully pull skin off chicken breast and insert sage leaves. Sprinkle with salt and place chicken thighs on top of bok choy / fennel mixture. Place uncovered in oven and bake for 40 minutes or until chicken reaches internal temperature of 150°F.
5. Serve chicken breasts atop bok choy / fennel mixture and sprinkle with fresh thyme.

CHICKEN BAKED IN CARROT SAFFRON SAUCE

MAKES 4 SERVINGS

1/2 cup olive oil

2 pinches saffron

4 medium carrots

1 1/2 teaspoons salt, divided

Juice and zest of 1 lemon

4–6 chicken thighs (bone in and skin on)

1. Preheat oven to 350°F.
2. Warm olive oil and saffron in saucepan for 10 minutes. Let cool for 10 minutes.
3. Roughly chop carrots and add to blender. Add saffron-infused olive oil, 1 teaspoon salt, lemon zest, and 1 tablespoon fresh lemon juice and blend until smooth.
4. Place chicken thighs in cast-iron skillet or oven-safe pan small enough so that the carrot sauce will cover chicken thighs. Sprinkle with half teaspoon of salt. Bake uncovered for 50 minutes. Serve warm.

CONCLUSION

The riches of deep loving
are yours.

♥

WE'VE ALL HAD SAD and difficult experiences in life. It doesn't
really work to organize your life to try to skirt difficulty. Your
relationship to your illness matters, however, and ultimately difficulty is
here for your benefit to help you grow and gain wisdom. I believe it is
useful to establish real skills to assist you when difficulty does arise instead of trying to push it away. Many times when tough situations occur,
we think, *Oh no. Not this.* You may often feel like this, too—when you
feel yourself starting a flare or when you eat the wrong food. When you
go to the doctor for the test results and you are worse than before. When
you are doing The Loving Diet 110 percent and still waking up with aching joints. Or when you feel tingling in your arms and fingers and wonder if something serious is happening in your body. Autoimmune disease
can be a lonely struggle that no one seems to relate to. But those are the
places that have healing, because every single one of these struggles is
asking you to believe in yourself. It's not easy, but when that pain or
struggle strikes and you're buried in stress and sadness, remind yourself
that it is going to be okay. And when you do, when you believe yourself
worth believing in, healing and miracles take place.

If you believe the premise that what we are is what we attract, then
if we are against things in our life, like our bodies or our diagnoses, we
attract againstness. Not that I am going to propose that is a *bad* place to

be. It takes engaging in againstness to ultimately teach us to choose cooperation, so it has tremendous value. No matter which way you choose, you will have the opportunity to keep choosing until you come into cooperation with your soul, which is the path of love. Againstness can show up as feeling like we're not getting answers, or it can be an internal feeling of disappointment or frustration, or that life isn't working out very well. That's why how we position ourselves is important, because what we are on the inside is what we attract on the outside.

As you come into cooperation with your life, and as you build skills to trust your life more deeply, the idea that it is loving wisdom pushing your life forward when difficulty does arise will provide you with a larger vantage point to operate from. A vantage point that helps you make more sense of difficulty. The more you invest in that love, the more your life is going to meet you with love. Illness is one way that life tries to show us wisdom, and when we trust the wisdom, when we trust the messages, when we trust that the illness is coming forward to teach us something, then life unravels itself to re-ravel itself in a different way that's more in alignment with our own heart. Illness is here to wake you up to something.

It's kind of like a baseball team. When you train to become a better baseball coach, then you get a better baseball team. As your new team comes together though better coaching skills, the old team can seem like it's falling apart or falling away. It can be startling and a little scary to say good-bye to old players and feel unsure to trust the new players, but the more you're continually investing in this process and then trusting, you can have an awareness that, when things in your life dismantle themselves, it's just a symptom of things coming back together in a way that's going to work better in your life, and illness is just a symptom of that. Illness is the vehicle and loving is the tool for getting the life you want.

Illness is a powerful medium for wisdom, and when you decide you want to use illness as a gift giver, life opens itself to you. Once you decide that, once you choose it, once you're trusting, then your life can shift. Illness is a cleverly disguised nugget of wisdom about increasing loving in your life, getting the life you want, and awakening to the truth that you deserve those riches in life. Illness is a vehicle to get you to the loving place inside of yourself. In order to do this, I suggest to love what's present, love the illness, love your circumstances, and take 100 percent responsibility for your life. Then everything you experience is simply a means to get you to a deeper wisdom.

Even if you don't know what the outcome is going to be, you have the opportunity to make the decision to work with your circumstances. That can create immediate change. Prayer, mindfulness, working with your circumstances, reframing beliefs, releasing beliefs, and forgiveness all place you in an immediate state of cooperation with your life. It's an internal cooperation, with you making the decision to buy into that belief. And all of those techniques are more of an awakening action and less of a doing action. Awakening to cooperation is an aligned state of affinity. There, in the aligned, cooperative state, reality can present itself on the outside of you in a cooperative aligned state. Peace is a side effect of going into cooperation with your life, trusting your life, and actively searching for the blessings. Peace is a side effect because when you trust your life 100 percent (which means trusting the illness, too), then you're placing yourself straight into alignment. Loving what is present is the quickest way of going into alignment with your life.

I did this and made an investment into a deeper place than diet, supplements, lab work, doctors, and stress management can go. I made an investment in myself that I could face a difficult, sad thing. I did not push away the dread, or the sadness, or the difficulty. I welcomed them all in as tools to help me uncover a valuable lesson of wisdom being presented to me: to choose the most loving path for myself. This is the surest place of healing. Run toward what ails you. It is the quickest way through it, and if you move beyond the good and bad of it, there are nuggets of gold for you. Gather the nuggets of gold even if through tears of sadness. If you are sad, know from the deepest place inside your soul that you are not alone on this journey and love will catch you, always and forever, if you let it. And when it catches you, consider that it may not look like what you want or think. There may be sadness. There may be suffering. There may be illness. There may be heartache or uncomfortable change. Trust that. Trust the unwinding the universe is doing. Because the investment in loving means you are guaranteed to be put back together again in a new way that will serve you better. That is the deal with love. As you choose it, it chooses back. Being born on the planet gave you a ticket to this resource of loving that will never expire. And that is The Loving Diet. Choose it. Choose you. Choose that you can do this. Choose the loving inside yourself that is the strongest and most solid resource you have. And stay fierce in your loving.

THE LOVING DIET PRACTITIONER

If you are interested in working with a Loving Diet Practitioner or learning how to become trained in this compassion-based health coaching, please visit my website, www.aiplifestyle.com.

Also on my website are resources for more information about working with me directly, Autoimmune Paleo recipes, and upcoming speaking engagements and workshops that present The Loving Diet.

BEYOND DISEASE

Does The Loving Diet work for issues besides autoimmune disease? Absolutely. It is a perspective you can take for the whole of your life. In fact, I used The Loving Diet principles I put forth in this book to heal my own heartbreak. Any life event or situation that creates struggle, suffering, or the loss of joy can benefit from The Loving Diet approach. Illness and disease is simply the vehicle you are using to gain wisdom. We all have our own unique vehicles of maximum wisdom-giving events: death, heartbreak, job loss, betrayal, and illness, to name a few. Love is the only energy in the universe that cannot be controlled or manipulated, so it makes sense to use love as a powerful healing tool. Love is also not bound by time or space so it is instantaneous. Love is here for you at this very moment, waiting for you to call upon it. It is the language of your own heart asking you to awaken to it. Love is the journey our souls are here to take. Illness is your road to grace. And when you choose grace and love, never will there be a moment of being alone. Always and forever.

RESOURCES

LABS AND LAB WORK

Here is the lab work I recommend clients ask their doctors to run. You can get this run yourself through www.directlabs.com. This panel is called their APEX-5 Panel.

Comp Metabolic Panel w/ eGFR
CBC w/ Diff
C-Reactive Protein
Ferritin
Hemoglobin A1c
VLDL
TIBC
% Iron Saturation
Serum Iron
Sed Rate
TSH
T3

T3 Uptake
T4 Thyroxine Total
T4 Thyroxine Free
Reverse T3
Free T3
Uric Acid
25 Hydroxy Vit D
Anti-TPO
Anti-TGB
Homocysteine
Standard Urinalysis

Stool and SIBO Tests

Genova Diagnostics
www.gdx.net
Genova Labs GI Effects 2200
SIBO Breath Test

Doctor's Data
www.doctorsdata.com
Comprehensive Stool Analysis w/ Parasitology

Commonwealth Labs
http://hydrogenbreathtesting.com

DiagnosTechs
www.diagnostechs.com
Cortisol Testing

BioHealth Lab
http://biohealthlab.com
Cortisol Testing

DIY Lab Testing Online

www.accesalabs.com
http://directlabs.com Immune Testing

Cyrex Labs
www.cyrexlabs.com

PRACTITIONERS & HEALTH EXPERT RESOURCES

Dr. Datis Kharrazian, DHSc, DC, MS, MNeuroSci, FAACP, DACBN, DABCN, DIBAK, CNS
http://thyroidbook.com
http://brainhealthbook.com/datis-kharrazian
http://drknews.com
Dr. Kharrazian's thyroid practitioner locator: www.thyroidconnections.com

The Institute for Functional Medicine
www.functionalmedicine.org

Carrick Brain Centers
http://carrickbraincenters.com

Dr. Mark Pimentel, MD
www.cedars-sinai.edu/Research/Research-Labs/Pimentel-Lab

Linda Clark, MA, CNC
http://uwanutrition.com

Dr. Allison Siebecker
www.siboinfo.com

Ryah Nabielski, MS, RDN
http://ecologicalnutrition.com

Dr. Andrea Rosario, DC, DACNB
www.flihealth.com

Charmayne Kilcup, PhD
http://charmaynekilcup.com

Holly Marshall, nutritional practitioner
www.hollymarshallnc.com

Jessica Flanigan, nutritionist, The Loving Diet founder
www.aiplifestyle.com

MEDITATION

UCLA Mindful Awareness Research Center
http://marc.ucla.edu/body.cfm?id=22

Chopra Center Meditation
https://chopracentermeditation.com

Eckhart Tolle
www.eckharttolletv.com

Omega Institute
www.eomega.org

ACKNOWLEDGMENTS

I would like to thank my teacher, Robert Waterman, EdD, LPCC, who for me is the physical embodiment of grace and love. Words fall short for the appreciation I have for such a wise teacher. I sit in honor of you. Thank you.

To all the brave souls who have transformed my life in the form of heartbreak, heartache, struggle, and loss. Thank you. While I may have shed tears of sadness with or about you, it is you who paved the way to widen and grow my heart. Truly you have helped me love this journey. I will always love all of you.

To my daughter, Mae, who saw me fall apart and come back together again in a new way. Your fierce loving is what I aspire to.

My twin sister, Danielle, who set me on the path of Autoimmune Paleo through your own teacher of autoimmune disease, and all the days you told me I could do this and really meant it. Thank you for being my dear twin and for our spiritual journey we support each other on.

My girlfriends who never gave up on me in my darkest moments. You watched me unravel and believed I would be okay. Trisha Graham, Jilan Glorfield, Nikiya Schwarz, Raelynn Noel, and Kate Elliott. You all are my earth angels. Thank you.

To Daniel Flanigan and Nadia Yavorsky for teaching me that peace is a place inside myself. Thank you both for letting our family grow into a new and beautiful unit.

To Stephanie Krikorian, who pulled out her magic fairy wand and wove *The Loving Diet* together in a coherent, beautiful form. Your humor, brilliance, and razor-sharp wit was a joy to experience. I can't wait to do it again.

To my editor, Lara Asher: When you said you do the Whole 30 program, I knew we would get along and knew you would totally get my big picture. And you did. Thank you for being such a kind and wonderful listener.

To my publisher, Post Hill Press, for appreciating that Paleo and Mindfulness have a home together.

To my clients, your courage and bravery allow me to wake up each day excited to change the nature of health care. You are the bravest of the bunch. May each time it appears you are slipping through the cracks of the health-care system deliver you to the new place of health and healing. I humbly walk in love with all of you.

ABOUT THE AUTHOR

Jessica Flanigan is a nutritionist specializing in the Autoimmune Paleo Diet. She is a leader in the Autoimmune Paleo movement, and she has seventeen years of experience as a functional clinical nutritionist. She has a decade of experience in the mind-body field. She developed The Loving Diet™ after working with chronically ill clients who were searching for deeper meaning through their illness. It is based on principles of Noetic Field Therapy™, functional clinical nutrition, and her own decades-long nutrition intuition practice. The Loving Diet incorporates the basic principle that any conflict in our life or physical body that comes present is meant to bring us closer to our divine nature. Through releasing outdated patterns of belief that no longer serve us, we align with cooperation inside of our self so that life and reality then form around us congruent with cooperation. Health and abundance come forward more rapidly in that state and produce a more joy-filled life. In the end it is changing how we feel about our circumstances rather than changing our circumstances that can produce healing results. She teaches her clients to use everything to their advantage, including physical illness. Flanigan maintains a private practice seeing clients via Skype for both Autoimmune Paleo nutrition and The Loving Diet program. She also conducts The Loving Diet workshops and professional trainings around the country. She lives in Northern California, and you can visit her on the web at aiplifestyle.com.